CELEBRATE YOUR SEASONS

CELEBRATE YOUR SEASONS

Inspirational Devotions to Progress in Love and Grace

Gabriella D. Filippi

Hamilton Books
A member of
The Rowman & Littlefield Publishing Group
Lanham · Boulder · New York · Toronto · Plymouth, UK

Copyright © 2011 by
Hamilton Books
4501 Forbes Boulevard
Suite 200
Lanham, Maryland 20706
Hamilton Books Acquisitions Department (301) 459-3366

Estover Road
Plymouth PL6 7PY
United Kingdom

All rights reserved
Printed in the United States of America
British Library Cataloging in Publication Information Available

Library of Congress Control Number: 2010939660
ISBN: 978-0-7618-5453-1 (paperback : alk. paper)
eISBN: 978-0-7618-5454-8

∞™ The paper used in this publication meets the minimum
requirements of American National Standard for Information
Sciences—Permanence of Paper for Printed Library Materials,
ANSI Z39.48-1992

Praise for
Celebrate Your Seasons

"Life is daily and the seasons regular. In *Celebrate Your Seasons*, Gabriella Filippi provides a guide on how to have a love relationship with God in every season. The book is not only inspirational, but practical."
                    GARY CHAPMAN
        Author of *The Five Love Languages* and *Love as A Way of Life*

"An inspirational devotional read with a deep connection to the wisdom of Solomon and the gritty reality of everyday life. Gabriella leads us into the quite space of God's creation, not pressurizing but easing the reader into restorative contemplation. *Celebrate Your Seasons* would be a worthy companion throughout each season."
            Reverend WILLIAM VAN DER HART
                    St. Peter's West Harrow, London

"Like a friend who walks through life with you, *Celebrate Your Seasons* holds your hand through the turns on the winding road of life. Lessons we all need to be reminded of daily . . . insights into the small things and large things . . . Gabriella wraps these truths around us like the loving arms of a mother's touch. Invite her on your journey!"
                    CELIA WHITLER
                    Singer, songwriter, author

"Gabriella Filippi's thirteen week devotional inspires and empowers readers to live a fuller, richer, Christian life. Each day's writings include Scripture, a reflection, questions, and a meaningful quote to stimulate thought provoking discussions and personal action. *Celebrate Your Seasons* is well-written, readable, and can be used individually or as a springboard for small group study."
                    MARY K. DOYLE
            Author, four books, including *Mentoring Heroes*

"*Celebrate Your Seasons* enables the individual to take a new pathway of life with effectiveness and joy. Who would not be better prepared to meet the challenges of daily thinking and living than the reader of this book! It ushers us into a land of self-discovery and self-actualization which effects progress. It affords conscious worth, empowering the reader to surmount obstacles. The book has the intent to transform: it does."
                DR. JOAN FRANKLIN SMUTNY
    founder and director of The Center for Gifted, an affiliate of National-Louis University; author and editor of sixteen books, with the latest,
                Differentiating for the Young Child

Devoted to my Heavenly Father:
Master and Beacon,
who has each moment positioned
as it is meant to be.
You give us breath and take it away.

Dedicated to my earthly father, Walter,
who led as he followed the Lord.
Miss you incredibly.
We never fully realize what we have
until it's gone.

Contents

Foreword

Preface

Acknowledgements

Introduction

God's Faithfulness Throughout the Seasons

Week One	Seek Purpose	
	A Time to be Born and a Time to Die	
Week Two	Sow and Reap	
	A Time to Plant and a Time to Uproot	
Week Three	Restore To Health	
	A Time to Kill and a Time to Heal	
Week Four	Encourage	
	A Time to Tear Down and a Time to Build	
Week Five	Freshen Up	
	A Time to Weep and a Time to Laugh	
Week Six	Celebrate Passion	
	A Time to Mourn and a Time to Dance	
Week Seven	Thought, Word, Deed	
	A Time to Scatter Stones and a Time to Gather	
Week Eight	Forgiveness and Acceptance	
	A Time to Embrace and a Time to Refrain	
Week Nine	Exalt, Glorify, Praise	
	A Time to Search and a Time to Give Up	
Week Ten	Give and Receive; Bless and Be Blessed	
	A Time to Keep and a Time to Throw Away	

Week Eleven	Broken but Willing ~ Reduce and Grow A Time to Tear and a Time to Mend	99
Week Twelve	Aspire To Inspire A Time to be Silent and a Time to Speak	109
Week Thirteen	Love and Be Loved A Time to Love and a Time to Hate	119
Closing Moments	Seasons A Time for War and a Time for Peace	128
Deliverance	The Prayer	130
Notes		132
Appendix		133

Foreword

Celebrate Your Seasons is an opportunity to create a personal relationship with God one day at a time and transform our lives through love, understanding, and personal humility.

There is a propensity among humans to want to see into the future and then after seeing what awaits us, manipulate every event that leads up to the event, good or bad. The flaws in our thinking are that the future will be exactly as we imagined or that nothing unforeseen, good or bad, is going to happen that changes everything. There's even a third possibility that is the most neglected opportunity of all. The idea that there could be an even better outcome on its way that's beyond what we are capable of imagining right now.

But if we can't imagine what it is, how do we get to it? We rush past so much of what is right in front of us and only remember later how good it was and wistfully wish for the time to come back to us.

However, there is a better way and it always starts with a recognition that we are loved by God in this moment and can choose to turn to Him for our answers.

Gabriella Filippi offers readers a guide that takes us through each season of building a better relationship with Him and along the way building a better relationship with others and ourselves.

Celebrate Your Seasons is being offered to the public at a unique time in our history when many people have been brought to their financial knees after a heady spree of buying for the sake of owning. We are ready to listen to an old idea that's new to us and readers will be grateful for an opportunity to be reminded that God loves us without end and without conditions. We are free at last to be ourselves as we are in this day and then to be of service to Him and to others.

If you are feeling empty, have lost your financial standing, or just want to bolster your ongoing relationship with God, *Celebrate Your Seasons* is another guide to light the path.

Martha Randolph Carr
Nationally Syndicated Columnist and Author of *A Place to Call Home*

Preface

There is a time for everything,
And a season for every activity under heaven:

A time to be born and a time to die,
A time to plant and a time to uproot,

A time to kill and a time to heal,
A time to tear down and a time to build,

A time to weep and a time to laugh,
A time to mourn and a time to dance,

A time to scatter stones and a time to gather them,
A time to embrace and a time to refrain,

A time to search and a time to give up,
A time to keep and a time to throw away,

A time to tear and a time to mend,
A time to be silent and a time to speak,

A time to love and a time to hate,
A time for war and a time for peace.

Ecclesiastes 3:1-8

Experience God's faithfulness through every season. Wise King Solomon discovered this late in his life, c. 935 B.C., after trying it all. Solomon, son of King David and the presumed author of Ecclesiastes, asked the same powerful questions that we ask today, and made identical statements to ancient language, as established in the Dead Sea Scrolls.

The Ecclesiastes outlook that "everything is meaningless" has been termed pessimistic or discouraging. These verses actually present the opportunity to teach us that difficulties wake us up, obstacles grow our spirit, and obstructions bring us closer to God.

God gave Solomon great knowledge to be wiser than all, yet Solomon discovered what we have sensed to be true throughout time: that we find our purpose through God, in God, and with God. Life cannot be lived apart from our Creator, the Author of Life. The God of purpose has each season planned and every breath accounted for.

Acknowledgements

Thank you with all my heart to my dearly loved family, friends, and even friends of friends whose prayers, support, and encouragement elevated this project from vision to reality.

Gratitude to the writers and thinkers whose insight and inspiration I have quoted in this book, to season more people's lives with their virtuous wisdom. Through extensive research, necessary reprint permissions were obtained. My apologies if any were missed, and modifications will be made accordingly in a subsequent edition.

The following authors, their agents, and publishers graciously granted permission to include and reprint by permission respective quotes and/or excerpts: Dr. Gary Chapman, Doc Childre, Disney family for Roy Disney, Chrissy Ogden Marsh, Sara Paddison, Norman Stone for the W. Clement Stone estate, and Pastor Phillip M. Way.

I express gratitude to the publishers and editors at Rowman & Littlefield Publishing Group, especially Bethany Blanchard, Brian DeRocco, Samantha Kirk, Victoria Koulakjian, and Sarah Stanton.

Special thanks to world leaders Reverend William Van der Hart and Pastor Daniel Darling.

My sincere appreciation to the various authors, artists, editors, and colleagues who helped raise this project: Kathy Born, D.C. Brod, Martha Randolph Carr, Dr. Gary Chapman, Mary K. Doyle, Sally Edmondson, Jamie Haith, Mary Harmon, Manette Monteclaro, Debbie Ross, Mo Sullivan, Dr. Joan F. Smutny, Celia Whitler.

Dear Martha, I've thanked God many times over for sending you. Your forethought urged me to press on, let go, or *breathe* ~ all at appropriate moments. God surely has you.

Thank you dearly, Mama ~ despite your rigorous journey these past two years, you cheered and encouraged me, and championed my cause, especially through my final months of writing and compilation.

Through my three treasured heartstrings, Lucas, Natalie, and Marisa, have I come to know unconditional love and grace . . . God's greatest gifts in my life.

Grateful to you, Craig . . . through Him we continue to grow in grace and love.

My sincere desire for you, beloved friends, is to be blessed through the Scriptures and words penned in this book and to *Celebrate Your Seasons*™ each and every day.

Introduction

Seasons during the calendar year, the years of our lives, and circumstances pulsate with a natural rhythm yet changes in these seasons often present distressing uncertainties. Just as we can depend on winter, spring, summer, and autumn's rotation, we experience steady increases of noteworthy episodes in our lives as we mature; ones that produce sorrow and joy, pain and pleasure. When each period ends, a new one begins, filled with different opportunities and challenges. We have choices in direct proportion to our willingness to grow as to how we will mature through the different stages. With slow, careful consideration we can grow to appreciate the four seasons of anticipation, exaltation, revelation, and tribulation as spring opportunities, summer excitement, autumn epiphanies, and winter complexities. These passages comprise more than our calendar year; they make up our daily lives. Each season holds a purpose; each purpose has its season.

Celebrate Your Seasons weaves the Scripture from Ecclesiastes 3 into daily themes over the course of thirteen weeks, the breadth of a season. Themes shape questions that incite thoughts, exercises, meditations, and prayers to feed the mind, body, and spirit. *Celebrate Your Seasons* offers inspiration and deeper insight to the understanding and refining of the self in relation to the overall purpose of existence. Changes are then embraced rather than resisted.

We may encounter and live multiple seasons simultaneously. Each episode presents its own opportunities for growth ultimately moving us towards completion, as humans created by God in His likeness (Genesis 1:26.) We were destined to fully experience each season, in every sense of the word, as it unfolds. As we grow, we experience guidance so that we can lose what is temporary in order to gain what is eternal by entrusting the God of the Universe who imparts plans that he has for us—plans for good and not for disaster, to give us a future with a hope—His promises in Jeremiah 29:11. We learn to celebrate each season, progress, and grow.

To attain harmony in this earthly world around us, essential peace begins with the world inside of us, commencing with self-awareness and the refinement of our morality. We learn to grow closer to God daily so that we may know Him better, as we learn to grow and know ourselves. Progressively, we then experience a more fulfilling relationship and through the seasons we are seasoned. We appreciate the inherent time and intended purpose for everything, which is the Ecclesiastes 3:14 vow: "I know that everything God does will endure forever, nothing can be added to it and nothing taken from it. God does it so that men will revere Him." God surely meets us in every season.

Apache Seasons

There once was a man who had four sons. He wanted them to learn to not judge things too quickly. So he sent them each on a quest to find a pear tree that was a great distance away and study it. The first son went in the winter, the

Introduction

second in the spring, the third in summer, and the youngest son in the fall.

When they had all come back the father called them together to describe what they had seen. The first son said the tree was ugly, bent, and twisted. The second son said it was covered with green buds and full of promise. The third son said it was laden with blossoms that smelled so sweet and looked so beautiful, it was the most graceful thing he had ever seen. The last son said it was ripe and drooping with fruit, and was full of life and fulfillment.

The man told his sons they were all right, because each had seen but one season in the tree's life. "You cannot judge a tree, or a person, by only one season," he told them. "The essence of who you are, and the pleasure, joy, and love that come from your life, can only be measured at the end, when all the seasons are fulfilled."

You are in the right season

Seasons change, but you are right where you need to be now. If you give up when it's winter, you will miss the promise of spring, the beauty of summer, and the fulfillment of fall.

We journey through life just once. Relish breakthroughs in spring, absorb the abundances of summer, harvest realizations in autumn, and learn from challenging lessons and strength-gathering rest during winter. Experience fullness in each type of season—during the year, in circumstances, and while growing older. Acknowledge their splendor and the consecrated moments of time in which they arrive. However, be willing to also experience true growth, which necessitates submission; surrender to God's plan as each season unfolds. As we relinquish personal purpose to our Creator, we walk fearlessly in faith toward a new self, complete with God's almighty grace and blessing.

In this inspirational devotional, we will take a closer look at daily life to alter attitudes that prohibit growth, and make decisions about life's direction and intent based on each topic. Through a process of slowing down and stillness, quiet contemplation and thoughtful reflection evolve so we can explore, express, and expand the thoughts, feelings, and desires on a daily basis. Along the way we can take notes, sometimes written, but more often they will remain in our hearts, heads, and souls. We are on a journey to unravel our genuine selves so that our identity that we keep private matches the image we present in public. As soon as we routinely work on trueness to our real self, we capture and cultivate the inherent self, a higher character, the intentional image of our Creator. Travel lightly and grow daily by meditating on God's purpose for you and His world.

The eye of the season

We make adequate preparation when we see a storm in sight or hear news of its coming. We go indoors, close any open windows, and listen to the forecast. But there are gales and outbursts that approach without warning—no thunder, lightning, or even a drop of rain—when we just don't have enough time to prepare. These occurrences have the potential to set us back. Stunting storms signify frustration, aggravation, temptation, and lamentation.

The eye of a storm is the calm weather at the core of a powerful cyclone, surrounded by soaring thunderstorms and intensely severe conditions. While storms typify exterior conditions, the same can occur internally, as we strive for peace amidst disarray. With each day of every season of diverse circumstances, visualize serenity inside the storm ~ rest in the eye of the season. As each story or daily meditation unfolds, you are challenged to enter into quiet contemplation to regain perspective concerning storms that surround you or pinnacle moments that elevate you, finding wisdom and strength in a solid foundation: the opening Scripture. Utilize the verse as a focal point, drawing reference to it as you seek solitude or moments of silence, reason through your thoughts, center yourself, pray, and then learn more about yourself as God reveals His love to you.

Commence

A time to be born. A time for renewal. A fresh start. A new beginning. We are born new. Whole. Unique. Unscathed. Fresh. Full of endless possibilities. And the possibilities are endless. Bitter cold and arctic days surround our cocoons where we nestle until a moment arrives for us to step out. Breathe. Begin.

We cart along possessions from one season into the next—some to sort, others to discard, still several more to embellish. Often we hang on to this *stuff*, unable to let go and resistant to change, year upon year and relationship after relationship with circumstance following circumstance. We can allow this to stifle us or we can resolve to grow despite the potential outcomes, and learn to celebrate each day of every season confident that its arrival is timely since our Creator fashioned us in His image. Increasingly, we attain awareness of a time to let go and a time to hold on, as He instills a passion in our hearts to guide our lives to completeness.

Our identities are established at birth. Yet, as we are molded and shaped by the values, ethics, and morals patterned in our roots, we can still grow and launch ourselves as a blend of nature, nurture, and belief. At times the lines are not distinct. However, the longer we live, the more apparent it becomes that our lives are stunning tapestries, skillfully fashioned in precise stages. If we can understand and enjoy the *process* more than the outcome, *growth* over routine, with a perpetual ambition to *give* instead of an expectation to *get* and *gain*, then we truly profit during life's journey.

Introduction

Each day is a new opportunity, as is the prospect of every year. Despite what occurred yesterday, let go of the past. Treasure people and places that present to you daily, for their significance is your unsolved mystery. Cleanse: meditate on the gifts of today, for tomorrow is uncertain.

There is a time for everything . . . this is your time.

God's faithfulness throughout the seasons

January—A time to be born—A time to die

Life's cycle: springtime joys often follow winter tribulations and mirror natural life events of birth and death. See beyond the obstacles to the opportunities ahead and launch or mature those character traits that are virtues. Expand and fortify the scope of God's purpose for you during this earthly journey.

February—A time to love—A time to hate

The greatest is love: an essential emotion to the eradication of inequality, to purge discrimination, to sear injustice. Loathe those negative, damaging traits enough to replace them with a powerful weapon—love—the vital tool for acceptance, healing, bonding, growth. Love is the supreme expression of thoughts, feelings, and actions.

March—A time to search—A time to give up

Go—grow: search for new prospects. Learn to recognize directions during the journey, and to heed warnings or acknowledge endorsements along the way. Ask, seek, and knock to receive answers in a relevant timing—God's timing.

April—A time to weep—A time to laugh

Rain and sun: while it is natural to adore sunshine, each season also presents precipitation. Rain likens to sorrow and weeping as sunshine to pleasure and laughter. The arid seasons necessitate water to refresh, restore, replenish, renew. Essential living water is vital every day of each season to support life.

May—A time to plant—A time to uproot

Transplant phase: every plant that was not reaped will be plucked up. Seasons arrive for entrance or exit from circumstances. Eliminate what doesn't work in life. There is a harvest time for all—a season to come into a full bloom and a time for things to die away.

June—A time to embrace—A time to refrain
Step closer or let go: strength of will is essential to healthy relations and experiences. They are threads that bind life. While essential goodness and unnecessary negatives surround life in tandem, discernment guides rightful thoughts and actions to engage or abstain.

July—A time to keep—A time to throw away
Save or discard: actions that are related to all the fibers that compose life's fabric. Decisions materialize as awareness shifts to action—when to persevere and when to surrender. While nothing lasts forever, life presents moments of gratification bestowed by God.

August—A time to scatter stones—A time to gather them
Forks in the road: clear a field or build a fence? Disassemble or assemble? Pursue an adventure or remain situated? Each activity is useful in its proper timing. Time and trials teach functional lessons and lasting significance.

September —A time to be silent—A time to speak
Rightful connection: times exist for discussion while other times necessitate refrain from chatter. Develop understanding for the timing and purpose that each type of communication and its implication presents.

October—A time to tear—A time to mend
The price of life: all is loss and gain. The push-pull of imminent loss or loss-recovery in the season of epiphany reveals the art of giving in, not giving up. Just as a mended garment is never quite the same as the original intact covering, splits recover in their appropriate time and in their own way.

November—A time to mourn—A time to dance
Life's tango: good times and bad compose the journey. Appreciation of purpose and significance to the light/dark, up/down, rejoice/grieve cycle of life changes perspective and attitude. A comprehensive, unending outlook can be developed to view the situations as they arise.

December—A time for war—A time for peace
Conflict avoidance: while evil lurks and seeks to destroy families and undermine nations, peace is the ultimate yet neglected goal. Wisdom reveals that the season of singing has come. The time and season has arrived to spread peace and good will throughout the entire journey, so that ultimately authentic completion arrives at the finish. True discovery rests in the awareness of the inherent purpose for life's seasons, where the end is just the beginning.

Introduction

Following His direction

God's purposes are incomprehensible, yet we trust His omnipotence and steadfastness in comfort, encouragement, protection, strength, and direction in every season during the span of our lives. Throughout our earthly journey, we are given opportunities to see how God's works are done to perfection, and we can attest to the beauty and harmony in all that is His, as we strive for a life that pleases Him. We receive opportunities to flourish and grow in His direction, with an awareness of intended purpose and timing to everything in God's overall scheme.

You are invited to log your principal moments of progression and growth in the Appendix. Additionally, each chapter concludes with a reflection page to journal how God leads you, how you follow Jesus, and how you hear the Holy Spirit each week. As you read: pray, meditate, write, bless, and be blessed.

Winter

Tribulation, woes

Evidenced by damp, bleak snows

Cold, stifling, icy

Dormancy abounds

Undisturbed stillness creeps in

Longing for freshness

© Gabriella D. Filippi

WEEK ONE

Seek Purpose

A time to be born

and

A time to die

Week One, Monday

Double Winter Doubts

"Everything that happens in this world happens at the time God chooses."
Ecclesiastes 3:1

Can't ever go back. Stark reality struck me like glacial, harsh, winter winds on my cheeks, days prior to the Christmas my father slipped away from his earthly existence. New Year's Day was the furthest from a feeling of happy for me. Was I living in a dream? How had life changed so rapidly? No more bear hugs, laughter, or walks and talks with the man I emulated. Doctor consultations in hospital corridors abruptly halted. Hospital emergency codes ceased. Now *goodbye* was final.

During this double winter season of my life, thoughts and emotions played tug-of-war as I vacillated between cleave or surrender. *Let go* echoed the voice to my ego. Would God's hushed, ever-present affirmation of His care transport me along a new journey? Could I remain content in the moment versus wedged in the past or perpetually expectant of the future? I searched with great intention.

Through seeking, answers arrive that can affirm and guide you to action. There are seasons in life where winter moments turn up as tests and trials even daily, which then require proper decision-making. Can you relate to this in your life? Have you experienced times when God allowed a winter so that He could bless you when He delivered a spring?

Whether life is on track or off course, today claim your life's intention. You may enter each season with old baggage, regrets, and downbeat tapes that play in your head. Peel away layers one day at a time so that the real you, then the renewed you, emerges. Liberate your life to a deliberate existence. Let go and grow in Christ. Take one day at a time and take time each day for a resolute rumination on God's purpose for you. Begin today to formulate a contract to be honest yet patient with yourself, asking, *what am I here for? What propels me forward? What will I do with the rest of my life?*

"But the plans of the Lord stand firm forever, the purposes of His heart through all generations."
Psalm 33:11

Week One, Tuesday

Nurture As You Are Nurtured

"So do not fear, for I am with you; do not be dismayed, for I am your God. I will strengthen you and help you; I will uphold you with my righteous right hand."
Isaiah 41:10

An old, seasoned tree has deep roots. Those roots were once new, small, and shallow. Nature establishes unique characteristics by which this tree grows and is recognized. While a tree may begin in a wild, primitive state untouched by civilization, when the tree is refined, nurtured, pruned, and cared for, it thrives.

Thoughts and feelings precede actions. We express our feelings as we nurture relationships with genuine care and love. In quiet moments as we contemplate or journal we allow time for meaningful thinking. During the stillness we release creativity and generate space for deep desires to root, and in doing so we step daily toward an intentional submission to fulfillment—God's way.

We can develop in the likeness of our Creator. He desires a full life for us. Complex emotional and intellectual attributes that determine a person's actions and reactions are established by nature, while nurturing plays a significant role in development. Did loving arms wrap around your shoulders when you felt the sting of your first fall or experienced the intense pain of your first heart break? Who nurtured you then? Who encourages you now? Do you desire to nurture in your life so that you can touch other lives? How can you cultivate great prayers along with celebrated thoughts, and cherish someone and something this day?

"Nurture great thoughts for you cannot go higher than your thoughts."
Benjamin Disraeli

Week One, Wednesday

Wisdom Beyond Years

"But the wisdom from above is first pure, then peaceable, gentle, reasonable, full of mercy and good fruits, unwavering, without hypocrisy."
James 3:17

My wise grandmother, Marianne, and I would visit for hours, baking and talking. Her compelling narratives vividly walked me through stories that revealed essential ingredients bestowed upon her in the face of trials while she remained focused on faith, devotion, and an undying will. My grandmother expanded my scope and excavated my conviction through these vivid anecdotes. I deeply desired to learn how she became seasoned through God's grace.

Though I gained education though Grandmother Marianne's accounts, I realized that ultimately we rely on our Provider for essential knowledge; knowledge that consistently precedes wisdom. We build understanding and amass good judgment with the hardships that furnish valuable life lessons, like a job loss, or worse, the loss of a friend. Knowledge accumulates in repeated learning, such as the times when we repetitively face incredibly similar situations—failing to realize that initially we didn't *get it*, only to painfully duplicate the process until we expectantly do *get it*. But we *get it* when we *apply* the word of the cross to gain wisdom. God's wisdom teaches us to recognize peace, truth, and discern good from evil. Our omnipotent Father, the Alpha and Omega, the beginning and end of wisdom, navigates us through each and every adversity.

How do you learn best: through deep discussions, trial and error, Scripture study, formal education, books? Do you eagerly seek opportunities to learn? Who helps you know and grow? How do you define wisdom? Do you seek God's wisdom for your proper discernment? Have you earnestly prayed for wisdom?

"There is no wisdom without knowledge."
Tom Braun

Week One, Thursday

Values Given, Values Made

"Therefore I tell you, do not worry about your life, what you will eat or drink; or about your body, what you will wear. Is not life more important than food, and the body more important than clothes? And why do you worry about clothes? See how the lilies of the field grow. They do not labor or spin."
Matthew 6:25, 28

When I lived in Sydney, Australia during my late teens, nearly all the clothing I possessed was stolen one day shortly after I hung them out on the wash lines to dry. At the outset, I was devastated and felt violated. Yet I learned a priceless lesson: Don't place too much value on things like clothes, or *rags* as our house manager affectionately termed them. Through this heinous act from an unknown thief, I realized they were just garments and now, carried off by someone who hopefully, indeed needed them. Perhaps the clothing provided cover for my temporary introverted personality. I could choose to get out and make friends by being a friend, and not allow change to displace my outgoing nature.

Possessions you value when you are young don't necessarily retain equal significance as you mature. Yes, certain items maintain their sentimental value, and yes, you grew up with a certain set of values that were perhaps placed upon you in earlier years. However, now you choose to establish the importance of value in relation to faith and morality, and make these the treasures in your life.

Do you put God first? Examine your valuables: what is number one? And subsequent to that? How do you determine the order? How do you feel when you lose something significant? Does it feel irreplaceable?

"It's not hard to make decisions when you know what your values are."
Roy Disney

Week One, Friday

Essential Ethics

"Not that I have already obtained all this, or have already been made perfect, but I press on to take hold of that for which Christ Jesus took hold of me. I press on toward the goal to win the prize for which God has called me heavenward in Christ Jesus."
Philippians 3:12, 14

Parents and caretakers regularly share essential values with their children. Values shape ethics, and in turn, ethics direct moral principles. *Make good choices* resonates all day long with the child who hears these as final words when they step out of the home each day. Choices define a person. And since thoughts precede actions, ethics serve as a barometer. Principles form our core beliefs and hence, our day-to-day acts, as well as provide commonalities we find in friendships, jobs, and other networks. Since principles are challenged daily, it becomes essential for us to listen to the Holy Spirit. Essential values and ethics have a Christian foundation, which makes it possible for the Holy Spirit to intervene, offering comfort and help to lead us toward Christ-like principles. We are encouraged to remain steady when our position is sound. An unspoken peace accompanies wise, ethical decisions, which ensue as we tune in to the Holy Spirit, the true inner barometer.

I have not yet reached my goal, and I am not flawless, but Christ has taken hold of me. So I keep on running and struggling to take hold of the prize, not satisfied until I cross that finish line of heaven.

Do you regard life with reverence, honoring serving and being more than having? Ethical principles may have sculpted our lives through those who raised us and with whom we grew up, but can we dive into our current belief system to discern which virtuous beliefs and actions will form a healthier family, a closer community, a stronger nation, a dedicated world in this moment?

"We have committed the Golden Rule to memory; let us now commit it to life."
Edwin Markham

Week One, Saturday

Morals Make Us

"If you do what is right, will you not be accepted? But if you do not do
what is right, sin is crouching at your door; it desires to have you,
but you must master it."
Genesis 4:7

What does it mean to do the right thing? In every aspect of our lives, we can strive to do the right thing. Without God morality does not exist. Societal laws differ and opinions vary on what is right, but for this reason God sent his son, Jesus, to show us what is right, how to make it right, ways to keep it right, and to right us when we're wrong, as long as we follow Him.

In all aspects of our lives, we can strive to do the right thing. A strong conscience ripens as we build morals, and vice-versa. At times, however, we select a certain path in hopes of instant gains. Through tackling the complicated decisions we discover that our values and principles shape our morals. Values, ethics, and morals are building blocks for character. And we find, as the saying goes, that past performance does not guarantee future returns. Our past performance may have actually demonstrated that choices made for short term reward yielded long term regret. Free will assigns us with the choosing. Sound, moral, Scripture-based decisions create a solid foundation for our principles and more importantly, gratify God. Our principles provide the standard which establishes a dogma for life.

What do you see in yourself and in life that you think is right? What about what you see as wrong? What guidelines or compass do you use? How do your morals support you and please your Maker?

"Moral choices do not depend on personal preference and private decision but
on right reason and, I would add, divine order."
George Basil Hume

Week One, Sunday

Surrender to Submission

"Submit to God and be at peace with him; in this way prosperity
will come to you."
Job 22:21

We do. We fix. We try. We make. We go. We return. This is life.

The pace gets rapid and choppy at times, doesn't it? Does the world attempt to have you conform to its ways of doing, constantly doing? The world may entice you to meld upstanding qualities, values, ethics, and morals to its often despondent, rebellious philosophy, while ultimately you choose to submit or not. Do we claim complete control of all, even the lives of others, while we could yield to ways beyond our own reasoning? Despite the world's persuasion and our internal struggle, we can still discard any principles that esteem power, prejudice, and pride. Chip away at this worldly grip for the higher cause, our Creator's seamless vision. Live *in* the world, but not *of* the world.

Complete submission entails gradual erosion of old ways in order to weave a delicate tapestry of new methods and manners intended for us by God—an uncomfortable surrender, especially for those of us who have decided we manage things just fine our way. After all, we realize that giving in requires giving up control. Submission calls for obedience, faith, and acceptance of the best plan for our lives, likely contrary to what we intended. We eventually learn that giving in does not mean giving up.

Have you had opportunities for submission, to release control and make greater gains, but ignored this calling? What results did you experience? Can you submit to the Master Plan?

"True strength lies in submission which permits one to dedicate his life,
through devotion, to something beyond himself."
Henry Miller

This Week

How God leads me . . .

_____
_____
_____
_____
_____
_____

How I follow Jesus . . .

_____
_____
_____
_____
_____
_____

How I hear the Holy Spirit . . .

_____
_____
_____
_____
_____
_____

WEEK TWO

Sow and Reap

A time to plant

and

A time to uproot

Week Two, Monday

Character Building

"But be very careful to keep the commandment and the law that Moses the servant of the Lord gave you: to love the Lord your God, to walk in all his ways, to obey his commands, to hold fast to him and to serve him with all your heart and with all your soul."
Joshua 22:5

An athlete's character develops in training, as they adapt to intense preparation. The athlete who yields to rigorous physical and psychological training today acquires dividends in the heat of an important event tomorrow. They know this approach best: daily discipline and thorough groundwork create support to their development. Junior building blocks amass to superior structure later, brick by brick, stone by stone, and step by step.

It is in looking back at our steps that we understand both the complexity in the climax and everything that led up to the event in our lives. Learned, life-changing moments that built and shaped our temperament likely occurred prior to goal completion, often while we walked through valleys. Because when we are willing to listen and absorb the experience of events that occur during challenging seasons, we realize these encounters frequently serve as a mirror to reveal the true persona, to shape and refine character flaws into personality strengths to season us spiritually. During tests, the temptation exists to turn back or to do nothing. Yet hardships produce strength of character. Character-builder opportunities march us onward, and we strive to do right, give our selfless best, and resolve to continue that forward walk through the valley. Step by step.

The Lord is pleased with uprightness. A character-builder begins with questioning self to grow integrity: *Does my internal quality complement my external temperament? Does the individual I encounter regularly at work, school, the store, or gym see me with consistent character? Am I steady and trustworthy?*

"Character may be manifested in great moments,
but it is made in the small ones."
Phillip Brooks

Week Two, Tuesday

Integrity and Authenticity

"I know, my God, that you test the heart and are pleased with integrity. All these things have I given willingly and with honest intent. And now I have seen with joy how willingly your people who are here have given to you."
1 Chronicles 29:17

I fall short day after day. Do you? Despite daily tests, I desire a life that leaves something of value for generations to come. Before I can do this, I earnestly seek to bring about refinement and conduct in myself so that I appear as polite and polished in public as in private. Once you and I value ourselves and work toward authenticity, we can proceed to grow a life shaped by integrity.

Accept yourself as you are: a unique, extraordinarily worthy person. When we have a keen sense of exactly who we are, we can strive to live accordingly—willfully honest and thus highly authentic. Despite the rigors of family and work obligations, extracurricular demands, travel, and long, erratic schedules, we can choose to not allow interferences in our conscious decision to live a life of integrity, to exist in this world beyond self, and to put aside self-importance for the higher cause, which is God's divine plan for our enhanced lives as we become better beings.

Do you pine for authenticity? Do you covet refinement to develop a life of integrity? If you do not already have a mentor, can you establish a relationship with someone faithful who can guide you towards a new life of sincerity and honesty?

"Have the courage to say no. Have the courage to face the truth.
Do the right thing because it is right. These are the magic keys to
living your life with integrity."
W. Clement Stone

Week Two, Wednesday

Respect All Around

"Give everyone what you owe him: If you owe taxes, pay taxes; if revenue, then revenue; if respect, then respect; if honor, then honor."
Romans 13:7

The Kindergarten playground provided a base-line for respect. Tugging a ball from a classmate's arms would have felt scandalous albeit we may have attempted it. Hence we learned the reciprocity of respect. Once we consistently provided respect, i.e., handed the ball over, it came back to us. Skilled at this game of give-and-take respect, we then used it often; until one too many days of disrespect.

Without respect for ourselves, how can we respect others and imagine others will respect us? Consequently, respect is not routinely given out, it is earned. Somewhere along the way though we decided to behave selfishly. As a selfish nature took over we lost respect—for others, but essentially for ourselves. Isn't it time for a little r-e-s-p-e-c-t?

Although the playground is bigger and more complex now, we realize that respect is based on commonalities that build its worth: faithfulness, equality, and truthfulness. With the use of respect we are more readily trusted and admired, reasonable and fair. We value other's opinions and they value ours. Importantly, we accept and respect ourselves unequivocally.

Do you respect yourself? How do you respect your Creator, planet, parents, teachers, coaches, mature individuals, persons of authority—essentially all those on your playground?

"Respect for ourselves guides our morals; respect for others guides
our manners."
Laurence Sterne

Week Two, Thursday

Unrelenting Hope

"For I know the plans I have for you," declares the Lord, "plans to prosper you and not to harm you, plans to give you hope and a future. Then you will call upon me and come and pray to me, and I will listen to you. You will seek me and find me when you seek me with all your heart."
Jeremiah 29:11-13

    We come to know God better when we witness how spring duly follows winter every year without fail. Challenging external winter seasons in our lives may mimic lengthy internal winters that we have endured. We question when the first signs of spring will actually arrive, and live with anticipation of color, foliage, and a warmer climate all temporarily resting just below the surface. Once we develop a deeper relationship with God we understand that during our winter tribulations He offers us rest to gain strength while preparing spring, even though we cannot see it or fathom it.

    Winter hardships can arrive during any season in the year. While winter is also a time of rest and energy replacement, when this season arrives it can easily deflate dreams and displace hope. A significant loss or death dislocates hope when we live a life without faith. Our Creator though assures us of a future filled with hope and goodness, in the face of suffering. Trials purify us. Optimism presents beyond the obstacles, so that we anticipate new opportunities. After winter arrives, faith is what instills hope in our unsettled world.

    God is good, all the time. All the time, God is good. And it's all good with God, who gives us hope and the realization that each moment and encounter is a blessing. Hope secured in deep faith invigorates, urges us to wish, plan, wait, and press on in expectation. Can you recall seasons of unrelenting hope?

"Never deprive someone of hope—it may be all they have."
H. Jackson Brown, Jr.

Week Two, Friday

Grace Refined Like Gold

"For it is by grace you have been saved, through faith—
and this not from yourselves, it is the gift of God."
Ephesians 2:8

The California Gold Rush peaked from 1849 to 1852. Plains farmers experienced a drought with seasons of poor harvests, which in turn meant modest money. Prospects of making vast amounts of money lured wagon loads of men, women, and children to California. People searched for, sifted, separated, and sanded precious metal pieces into valuable, durable, polished forms. Every person worked as hard as they could to help their families meet basic needs.

In its raw structure, grace matches gold. We are as strong as our weakest flaw, and we are all flawed. As we submit to character expansion and grow with God's grace, His acceptance helps us overcome our limitations. In grace we shift from a lack of refinement toward a steady devotion to improvement. He polishes us from raw form to beauty—with our submission and in His timing. We are beckoned and taught that with grace and in grace we have the power to endure heavy burdens and tribulations. And where sin increases, God increases grace all the more.

Grace increases our responsibility rather than reduces it. Grace is more real to us when we are faced with our weaknesses. God's grace strengthens our fragile links until we arrive at completeness. Just as gold diggers spent tedious hours refining precious metal, development in grace takes time. Have you realized grace in your life? Do you see God's grace in you?

"Grace is the absence of everything that indicates pain or difficulty,
hesitation or incongruity."
William Hazlitt

Week Two, Saturday

Pure J-O-Y

"The precepts of the Lord are right, giving joy to the heart. The commands of the Lord are radiant, giving light to the eyes."
Psalm 19:8

I gazed at the lemon tree in my sunroom and noticed how it leaned toward the light. Light: the source of nourishment that is needed to survive and thrive. The entire world benefits from sunshine. People seek light to function well and feel good. Similarly, those who exude light are a positive source and provide inspirational fuel often for others to survive and thrive.

At times we relate happiness with joy, using the terms interchangeably. While happiness is a choice and can exist merely momentarily, joy is deep-seated. Lasting happiness is independent of circumstances and is joy-centered living, a gift from the Spirit. Deep-rooted joy emotionally charges us and replaces temptations that divert energy in improper directions. Rather than permit a person or incident to deplete us of happiness, we can see beyond the situation and reach for inner joy, received from the Holy Spirit. The Spirit equips us to radiate when confronted with obscurity. When we place Jesus first in our lives, others next and ourselves last, we reflect light through deep-seated joy. The Spirit resides as light in us and we have the ability to typify beacons of joy in this world.

Visualize a joy-filled you. Imagine three personal moments of happiness stemming from a joy-centered life and detail the accompanying emotions. What choices that you make today will radiate your light to the world? How have you received the gift of joy that brought you peace and hope?

"JOY: Jesus, Others, Yourself."
Christian schools and churches around the world

Week Two, Sunday

Peace Within and Around From Above

"And the peace of God, which transcends all understanding, will guard your hearts and your minds in Christ Jesus."
Philippians 4:7

Create a visual picture of tranquility. As you feel your shoulders relax, perhaps you think of white sands, clear blue waters, and a cool breeze. Curled up on the couch with a good book may create your ultimate peaceful setting. Then again, cruising down the highway on a motorcycle or listening to a good country tune may bring harmony.

Now what happens once those peaceful moments evaporate? Can you find inner peace during mundane activities, stressful situations, and even times of sorrow? Like joy, we cultivate this lasting gift. Inner tranquility, rather than wealth and prestige mark true accomplishment and exude centeredness and harmony. Decisions are uncomplicated when we realize that the outcome ought to bring peace. Try not to figure anything out on your own. Ask God to speak to you and to guide you; then trust that He will. Be still. Listen for God's direction in all things, everywhere you go. God's Spirit instills true peace within us because His direction is peaceable. He is peace. Psalm 46:10 offers assurance of this: "Be still, and know that I am God."

Create a tranquil place. What does your snapshot of serenity look like? Can you retreat to this space, even if merely in your mind, when you experience unrest? When have you heard God's voice and felt pure peace? If God's voice is not present in your life, ask yourself, *have I been still long enough to hear it?*

"There is no way to peace; peace is the way."
A. J. Muste

This Week

How God leads me . . .

_____
_____
_____
_____
_____
_____
_____

How I follow Jesus . . .

_____
_____
_____
_____
_____
_____
_____

How I hear the Holy Spirit . . .

_____
_____
_____
_____
_____
_____
_____

WEEK THREE

Restore to Health

A time to kill

and

A time to heal

Week Three, Monday

Persistence and the Other Four P's

"Peace I leave with you; my peace I give you. I do not give to you as the world gives. Do not let your hearts be troubled and do not be afraid."
John 14:27

A time to kill and one to heal: God's judgment and His mercy. The eradication of old ways that prohibit growth and healing, urge a necessary step toward integrity, deeper faith, and changing harmful habits. Persistence and perseverance bound in prayer infuse patience and peace: the five P's to purpose. When we listen for guidance from the ultimate source of peace, God the Father, who works through Scripture, nature, and the Holy Spirit, and if we are constant and uncomplaining, we will benefit from the inner serenity that surpasses any form of human understanding. Once in tune with God's voice, we do not fret. We remain diligent, yet are not bent on working out every little detail. God works out the details for us.

When I decided to study and work overseas during my teen years, I applied to twelve universities in New South Wales. Not one accepted me. As I read through each negative response however, I remained patient, hopeful, and determined. In fact, the rejections provided fuel to pursue my ambition with deeper passion until I succeeded. Persistence and willingness to change my approach gave me the means to combat challenges and the necessary determination to advance the dream into reality.

The best way to fail is to quit. Instinctively concern looms while en route to accomplishing objectives when things don't go as planned, but worry can be displaced with unrelenting efforts directed by positive, thoughtful purpose rooted in prayer.

Do you welcome opportunities for persistence with positive thoughts and actions that assist in goal attainment? Are you steadfast in your efforts? When have you had the opportunity to displace worry with unrelenting peace, prayer, and patience?

"Knowing trees, I understand the meaning of patience.
Knowing grass, I can appreciate persistence."
Hal Borland

Week Three, Tuesday

Cling to Goodness

"They will celebrate your abundant goodness and joyfully sing of
your righteousness."
Psalm 145:7

Life requires regular housekeeping. There are times when we need to sift through useless, accrued possessions and purge. In doing so, we cleanse. We create order in our internal and external lives by keeping merely what is necessary and useful. As a result, we crave and select only the essential, we simplify life, and we expand our character and our circles by surrounding ourselves with others who also desire this same goodness. We release what no longer serves us in our homes, our work, and ourselves and recognize how to cling to the good.

Mother Teresa—Catholic nun, missionary, and Nobel Peace Prize recipient—the ultimate model of goodness, taught acceptance, selflessness, and humility as hallmarks of goodness. She held those inflicted with AIDS and kissed the hands of lepers. She demonstrated how good acts toward one another, no matter who it was, enabled a greater love for everyone and the ability to grow up in goodness. This type of goodness comes from God who works in us and through us to act according to his good purpose. When our actions match our words we model virtue, a quality that emphasizes people, not things, and keenly considers others as gifts. When we do deeds for others, we are doing great things for God. We move in closer to both relationships.

Doing good feels good. Have you experienced goodness recently as a donor or recipient? Have you had opportunities to utilize goodness? What do goodness and virtue mean to you?

"People are unreasonable, illogical, and self-centered. Love them anyway.
If you do good, people may accuse you of selfish motives. Do good anyway.
If you are successful, you may win false friends and true enemies. Succeed anyway. The good you do today may be forgotten tomorrow. Do good anyway.
Honesty and transparency make you vulnerable. Be honest and transparent anyway. What you spend years building may be destroyed overnight. Build anyway. People who really want help may attack you if you help them. Help them anyway. Give the world the best you have and you may get hurt.
Give the world your best anyway."
Mother Teresa

Week Three, Wednesday

Kindness Intercedes

"You gave me life and showed me kindness, and in your providence
watched over my spirit."
Job 10:12

Years ago, a teacher taught me the "pay it forward" concept of giving back through service that which I received from others. I understand it better now, having had opportunities to use it. If I extend myself with humanity, it works like money in the bank for future expenditures. When I or someone else needs an extension of kindness, it returns.

Pay it forward works especially well when least expected by the recipient. I experienced this one day while at the grocery store as I overheard a middle aged mother explain to her young son how they could not afford the treats he chose. A few minutes later, I rounded an aisle and ran into them again, seeing this mother count her money. As I headed toward the only open checkout lane, I now found myself behind them. *God is speaking to me here,* I thought, as I painfully watched this mother remove items from the conveyor belt so she could make her groceries meet her budget. After they paid their bill I quietly asked the clerk to ring up those items set aside from their order so that I might pay for them. *"You're paying for their groceries?"* the wide-eyed clerk asked. I nodded. Mother and son were exceedingly grateful, leaving me tearful but joy-filled. I invited them to carry on the theme with an extension of kindness for someone else later.

Kindness: a gift we are free to receive and a trait to refine. Even the smallest acts of kindness feel good and bless both giver and receiver. Acts of kindness repay the giver even before the act is done. Can you improve your world today with acts of kindness, applying compassion and sympathy? Why would we withhold kindheartedness from someone who needed it? Have acts of kindness come back to you, when least expected?

"Be kind, for everyone you meet is fighting a hard battle."
Philo of Alexandria

Week Three, Thursday

Walking in Faithfulness

"But the fruit of the Spirit is love, joy, peace, patience, kindness, goodness, faithfulness, gentleness and self-control. Against such things there is no law."
Galatians 5:22

Life gets confusing. Society tells us that if it feels good, do it. Yet if we are faithful and single-minded toward our commitments and primary purpose, we won't heed the advice. We'll think long and hard before we do anything that registers as doubtful. All too often in weak moments we falter and give in to convenience to attain satisfaction more easily, since our original game plan seemed to require too much work, allegiance, and devotion. During these moments, we need to ask ourselves: do we desire change that is built with faithfulness?

Our Creator desires the best for us, which entails a long, steady walk in faith toward Him and with Him. In order to arrive at fidelity, as Cicero pointed out over two thousand years ago, we step daily toward faith, trust, and confidence aimed at belief in what has not yet been seen. The enemy's attacks will taunt and tantalize us repeatedly, with attempts to destroy the good fruit we work diligently to produce. Each day is an opportunity to remain faithful to purpose and toward others, despite opposition.

When faith matures, we begin to realize divine purpose, alongside faithfulness to self and others. Truthful relations serve as a prerequisite for consistency and growth. During which season(s) has your faithfulness been challenged? In what ways can you grow in faithfulness while on this walk?

"Nothing is more noble, nothing more venerable than fidelity. Faithfulness and truth are the most sacred excellences and endowments of the human mind."
Marcus Tullius Cicero

Week Three, Friday

Guide with Gentleness

"A gentle answer turns away wrath, but a harsh word stirs up anger."
Proverbs 15:1

A certain peace coexists with the word *gentle*. When we allow matters to unfold rather than force them to take place, we have the ability to create a naturally milder approach to life. Gentleness permits the path of least resistance and greatest gain.

Relationship difficulties, work deadlines, travel commitments, illnesses, and erratic living conditions can all swiftly send us into an agitated mode. When situations become tense or too much has accumulated on those spinning plates, recall the kind and mild-mannered spirit waiting in the wings. We have a choice as to how we treat people or handle urgent situations. While our initial response to stressful encounters may be reactive, a proactive approach places us in a gentle mind-set and sets us free. Gentleness: positive thoughts, words, and actions to ward off roughness. When stressed, try composure by way of your gentle spirit.

Gentleness is another gift to develop throughout our lives. Rather than implying complacency, gentleness speaks to humbleness and humility. Much like grace, an element of bending takes place, with accompanying character development over time, in order for gentleness to work for us. We see things from another's point of view, and learn to consistently place others before ourselves. What gets in the way of your ability to provide gentleness when and where it is needed? Have you experienced gentleness today, as the benefactor or beneficiary? How can you offer gentleness this week?

"When you encounter difficulties and contradictions, do not try to break them, but bend them with gentleness and time."
Saint Francis de Sales

Week Three, Saturday

Friendship Completes Life's Circle

"If you have come to me in peace (friendship) to help me,
I am ready to have you unite with me."
1 Chronicles 12:17

    Without genuine friendships, life can feel empty and unfulfilled. A friend is someone who knows all about you and loves you just as you are; takes the appealing with the not so attractive. Companionship enhances the quality of life's experiences, carries us through difficulties, and benefits our emotional and mental well-being. Strong social networks even provide a protective effect against mortality. Sisterhoods and brotherhoods spanning the globe relish and uphold each other in this sacred bond called friendship. Friends hold us accountable, laugh with us, cry with us, keep our secrets, boost our confidence, share complexities, equalize intensities, and can still reflect what we see in ourselves. They are the co-partners of our dreams, coaches in our lives, protectors, companions, confidantes. While at times solitude is essential, ultimately, friendship completes life's circle.
    Friendship requires giving of self. C. S. Lewis describes the essence of friendship in *The Four Loves* as one in which each person is simply themselves, honest and open. A sincerely strong bond exists between two people who look at something together that is beyond or above themselves, often what originally formed the relationship.
    Could you imagine living without the enjoyment and extension of friendship? Are healthy relations important to you? How did your significant friendships evolve? Why have they flourished? How do you continue as a genuine, loyal friend during every circumstantial season? In what ways are your friends instrumental to your spiritual growth?

"We are born helpless. As soon as we are fully conscious we discover loneliness.
We need others physically, emotionally, and intellectually.
We need them if we are to know anything even ourselves."
C. S. Lewis

Week Three, Sunday

Owning Up

"Each one should test his own actions. Then he can take pride in himself,
without comparing himself to somebody else,
for each one should carry his own load."
Galatians 6:4-5

    A local newspaper gave an account of four older teenage males whose parents stepped in to take the blame for their sons' acts of violence that left one young man dead. Forty-three bystanders to this tragedy, mainly peers, neither attempted to stop the violence nor called for help despite nearly all of them having cellular phones that evening. The young men, facilitated by their parents, were not held accountable for their actions. Poor judgment, unfulfilled moral obligations, lack of self-control, and enablement—all point to a lack of adequate responsibility. What do we teach children if we step in to rescue them from their wrongful, harmful, and in this case, fatal acts? Will they gain responsibility?
    Life gets cluttered when we choose to get involved with family and friends. Yet responsible people by their trustworthy nature do what it takes without letting people down or taking over—tribulations included. Doing nothing is not an option. They know how to step up to the plate like a baseball player ready to make a hit. They *own it*. God wants to revive us out of our mediocre state, so that we step up to the plate: take charge, own what is ours, and become passionate, accountable, kind, and unselfish individuals who shape a brighter future—even, and especially, in the face of trials.
    Would your friends, colleagues, and family regard you as dependable, conscientious, and thoughtful to the outcome of actions? Do your close relations think of you when they need someone? In faithfulness?

"It is not for what we do that we are held responsible,
but also for what we do not do."
Molière

This Week

How God leads me . . .

How I follow Jesus . . .

How I hear the Holy Spirit . . .

WEEK FOUR

Encourage

A time to tear down

and

A time to build

Week Four, Monday

Care

"Be shepherds of God's flock that is under your care, serving as overseers—not because you must, but because you are willing, as God wants you to be; not greedy for money, but eager to serve; not lording it over those entrusted to you, but being examples to the flock. And when the Chief Shepherd appears, you will receive the crown of glory that will never fade away."
1 Peter 5:2-4

It's easy to become calloused to the needs of others when our own lives are so demanding. Why be bothered with caring for others when we are busy with our personal matters, our own set of problems? Care takes too much energy and time, both of which we have precious little extra. Then again, do we expect concern and sensitivity when *we* need it?

If you are someone who already has a serving heart, then you realize that when we serve others we serve God. We dish up and dole out because in serving we grow our hearts and prove love. We mature. When we develop a servant mentality, we gently, genuinely, guide others by changing coordinates. Everyone stands at the same level. Everyone assumes the same position. Everyone is important. Each one appears precious in God's eyes and God loves when we care.

Caring develops and sustains relationships that would dwindle if devoid of love and effort. Where do you recognize opportunities to care through service? Are you vested in relationships enough to nurture them to a higher level?

"Care is the actualization of love assumed. Care is the ingredient that keeps true friendship alive despite separation, distance, or time. Care gives latitude to another person and gets you past the dislikes and annoyances. Quite simply, caring sustains love."
Doc Childre

Encourage

Week Four, Tuesday

Compassion

> "... because his cloak is the only covering he has for his body. What else will he sleep in? When he cries out to me, I will hear, for I am compassionate."
> Exodus 22:27

Passion is literally at the root of compassion. As a social responsibility, compassion positions eagerness and genuine concern into your thoughts and actions towards others. Compassion surpasses sympathy and takes empathy to a deeper level. Daily we are presented with opportunities to be compassionate yet we may instead choose apathy or impartiality. What stops us or holds us back?

Several years ago, on a snowy Saturday morning in January, I received a call at home from a friend. A car had killed my friend's husband. He had actually survived the initial automobile collision, but immediately after his air bag deployed he stepped out of the car and was struck by an oncoming vehicle. My friend and I wept together over the phone for mutual comfort. I left everything and drove to her home to be with her and pray with her. At this time of distress and disbelief, I knew what she needed most was compassion from friends and family.

Like a warm blanket on a chilly day, compassion surrounds, calms, and soothes. Do you generously provide compassion when needed? Do you feel that unspoken peace when you passionately extend sympathy, empathy, concern, and kindness to someone? Have you recognized when God gives it back to you, and experienced that same calmness then? How can compassion guide your listening and hence, your actions?

> "Until he extends the circle of compassion to all living things, man will not himself find peace."
> Albert Schweitzer

Week Four, Wednesday

Humility

"... in the same way be submissive to those who are older. All of you,
clothe yourselves with humility toward one another, because,
'God opposes the proud but gives grace to the humble.'
Humble yourselves, therefore, under God's mighty hand,
that he may lift you up in due time."
1 Peter 5:5-6

Are you too proud or too afraid to be humble? Do you toot horns and voice team pride at a baseball game just as boldly as you praise yourself? Instinctive pride builds walls between people, goals, and growth. Release strongholds to create a clear view of an objective life without the ego to muddle relationships or circumstances, create missed opportunities for direction, or squelched curiosity.

High profile individuals often develop a low profile disposition likely learned through the abundance of seasons weathered in their lives. Skilled mentors partner with protégés to develop low maintenance, respectful, servant attitudes, and apprentice-to-professional aptitudes. The opportunity exists to strive for an appreciative and helpful nature to learn greater success.

Do you know how to be humble or do you know how to be proud? Are you humbled by strengths and gifted abilities while trained through weaknesses and areas necessitating improvement? Are willful and joyful obedience your tutors? Do you acclaim others?

"In reality there is perhaps no one of our natural passions so hard to subdue as
pride. Disguise it, struggle with it, beat it down, stifle it, mortify it as much as
one pleases, it is alive, and will every now and then peep out and show itself . . .
For even if I could conceive that I had completely overcome it, I should
probably be proud of my humility."
Benjamin Franklin

Encourage

Week Four, Thursday

Limits

"Do you listen in on God's council? Do you limit wisdom to yourself?"
Job 15:8

Limits span both ends of the spectrum. Somewhere in the middle of rigid limits and no limits rests healthy boundaries that maintain inherent focus and centered living. Drs. Cloud and Townsend exemplify limits as "boundaries" in their book, *Boundaries: When to Say Yes, When to Say No*. Boundaries are borders that allow people in but also reserve privacy. While God desires kindness from his children, our saying *yes* to everything and everyone often distracts us from His purpose for us. Like fences around a yard, borders protect our lives for harmony and stability, so we can discriminate who and what comes in and who and what stays out.

Boundaries abound: deadlines, office hours, budgets, speed zones, curfews, and more. Even thoughts and emotions have thresholds. We can establish margins and reduce the risk of placing too great of demands on others or ourselves. It's okay to say *no* to an optional activity, to pass on overextending yourself, and it is appropriate to take your own time out.

Consider your purposeful goals and visions, which have no restrictions. Intertwine them with God's purpose for you. Take time to meditate on where you need to establish healthy borders in your life and when to release the threshold in order to expand your purpose. Are you steadily growing? Do you pray for God to help you establish and maintain healthy limits?

> "To dream anything that you want to dream. That's the beauty of the human mind. To do anything that you want to do. That is the strength of the human will. To trust yourself to test your limits. That is the courage to succeed."
> Bernard Edmonds

Week Four, Friday

Cooperation

"It was for the sake of the Name that they went out, receiving no help from the pagans. We ought therefore to show hospitality to such men so that we may work together for the truth."
3 John 1:7-8

Team building is as essential in the workplace as it is on the playing field or in the home. Whether you are the giver or the recipient of cooperation, life is harmonious when all work is in concert. Burdens lighten as the load is shared. Cooperation, then, is a "team one" philosophy: When everyone participates fairly, all are on the same team and play with unified minds and hearts. Everyone wins, no matter the outcome.

A cohesive team attitude presents itself through trust and support. An offer to a frustrated store clerk by way of kind words or cooperative gestures, like a smile, funny story, or bagging your items, displays cooperation and defrays tension. Tension creates unnecessary stress and opposition. Opposition continually creates conflict, and conflict clashes with cooperation. If permitted, the vicious cycle continues.

As diverse and peculiar as individuals are, we need each other. God meant for us to live in community, and to establish trustworthy bonds that are dependent upon encouragement and effective communication. Unity among diversity makes life more interesting, and most especially when we support each other. Kinship circles strengthen through cooperation based on love. What is life if people are not here for each other? How do you view cooperation? Are you a team player or do you look out for number one? When have others aided you? How has that worked out for you?

"Now join your hands, and with your hands your hearts."
William Shakespeare

Encourage

Week Four, Saturday

Trust

"Trust in the Lord with all your heart and lean not on your own understanding."
Proverbs 3:5

Without genuine trust we teeter on a tightrope strung between our forged persona and our faithful person in waiting. Without trust we fall into a fake personality because we are too afraid to present the real self and no faith exists. To know who and when to trust is as central to stability as is too much or not enough trust. Yes, we need to trust each other. However, even people involved in a crime trust each other to some degree! Vital trust for positive growth is established through confidence in others for the right and reasonable acts and an equal if not deeper trust in ourselves.

During the initial years of our lives, we placed confidence in our caregivers to help us when we fell and to listen when we needed to talk. Without full comprehension, most of us learned to trust in early life. But if in those initial years you fell and no one came to your aid, you likely established distrust. As we grew older, we felt the same sting and despair of mistrust when we were lied to or we were let down in seemingly open, honest relations. We then learned how a lack of trust destroys, and that sadly not everyone is worthy of our reliance. While trust can come naturally and freely, discernment and trust act in concert, their conviction solidified over time.

In whom do you confide? You can place firm faith in your Lord and Confidant, above all. Can you trust Him before yourself, enough to discern and make the best decisions daily? How do those in your close circle, family and friends, view trust within the group? Do others have certainty and a firm belief in your character and in your reliability, ability, and strength?

"You may be deceived if you trust too much, but you will live in torment
if you don't trust enough."
Frank H. Crane

Week Four, Sunday

Modesty

"Humble yourselves before the Lord, and he will lift you up."
James 4:10

    With no compensation or ego-driven motive in mind, we can season the earth with talents bestowed upon us by our Creator. Place your finest, humble self forward, and you will be elevated. Salt away your best for the One who means the most to you. Humble people maintain an unassuming nature, open and honest, that attracts others like a magnet. Modest people are usually content with who they are, without airs. While wealth and prestige could easily shift their focus to self, they instead continually strive for the greater good, not defined by material possessions or social status. Modesty shuns the competition for worldly possessions. Contrary to popular belief, the one with the most possessions does not win; he may just have more to worry about.
    Modesty and meekness keep us humble when the temptation to boast knocks. Real appeal exists with those who don't flaunt their possessions and know their inner worth. Ancient wisdom from Lao-Tzu still rings true today: simply remain you in all areas of your life. You are the great being that God says you are! Strive toward the best you can be with a down-to-earth disposition as you measure up to God's intent, and raise the bar when He asks.
    Can you be yourself with just reverence for others? What does humility and meekness mean to you? Could you try going all day without using "I" in your conversations? Can you consider living outside yourself with careful discretion, present-day contentment, every day, God's way?

"When you are content to be simply yourself and don't compare or compete, everybody will respect you."
Lao-Tzu

Encourage

This Week

How God leads me . . .

How I follow Jesus . . .

How I hear the Holy Spirit . . .

Spring

Anticipation
Newness! The cycle begins
Darkness turns to light

Root, loom, and extend
With seeds the Maker has sown
Cultivate, go, grow

© Gabriella D. Filippi

WEEK FIVE

Freshen Up

A time to weep

and

A time to laugh

Week Five, Monday

Consistency by Way of Change

"Jesus Christ is the same yesterday and today and forever."
Hebrews 13:8

Mark Twain's play on words in his philosophy on change: the state of constancy equals change. Since change is steady, it is adaptation that establishes equilibrium. What a thorny task for those who desire to remain in their comfort zones.

In a game of tennis or golf, tradition seems to teach us that unfailing efforts usually win the match. The overall score depends on consistency—steady, powerful serves and return hits, or long drives and accurate putts. However, strategy sports, like tennis and golf, require that old habits change, often very quickly. Previously learned skills are constantly being unlearned in order to create a game that consistently wins using the newly acquired abilities. If we desire consistency in our core persona, the same applies—we must change. A consistent person is steadfast, unwavering, and open to unlearning negative qualities or qualities that no longer serve, to create stronger, more Christ-like traits. Change can create struggle, but through Christ as our mentor and coach, together with unwavering faith, we adopt development transformations yielding the character of a sincere Christian.

Are you willing to press the refresh button—to adapt in order to create consistency? Are you *yourself* time after time in diverse situations, such as at home, school, work, or in social situations? Who are *you* when no one is looking? Can you leave behind old traits and birth new, favorable, sincerely consistent ones?

"What then, is the true gospel of consistency? Change. Who is the really consistent man? The man who changes. Since change is the law of his being, he cannot be consistent if he is stuck in the mud."
Mark Twain

Week Five, Tuesday

Transformation Caterpillar Style

"Therefore, if anyone is in Christ, he is a new creation; the old has gone,
the new has come!"
2 Corinthians 5:17

Two caterpillars were walking down the sidewalk, eyes perched on a beautiful butterfly gliding through the air. One turned to the other and said, "You'll never get me up on one of those butterfly things."

Clearly risk avoidance isn't restricted to humans. Although often actively, consciously resisted, change is constant. Growth is optional. A butterfly does not begin as a butterfly. Metamorphosis occurs for the caterpillar without a conscious decision to change. The wonder of the butterfly life cycle lasts only a matter of weeks as it transforms from an egg, to a caterpillar, to a chrysalis, to another egg-laying butterfly. The butterfly sleeps inside the chrysalis until the intrinsic moment arrives for its entrance into the world as a transformed, elegant life form. While caterpillars drag their feet and focus only on eating and survival, the butterfly drifts with the wind and flies high above the ground to sense flowers and nature and to obtain provisions.

The human story is similar. We talk ourselves out of transformation and wrestle with change every step of the way. Either it entails too much risk, work, or our lineage and heredity dictate otherwise. Once we experience the beauty in the outcome, our perspective changes. New life *is* exciting.

We are all caterpillars with a butterfly's potential. Yet will we ever become butterflies if we remain caterpillars? Be patient with yourself and others as God's metamorphosis does its ongoing work.

"Nature often holds up a mirror so we can see more clearly the ongoing process
of growth, renewal, and transformation in our lives."
Mary Ann Brussat

Week Five, Wednesday

Walk Valleys, Climb Mountains

"More than that, we rejoice in our sufferings, because we know that suffering produces perseverance; perseverance, character; and character, hope."
Romans 5:3-4

All relationships bear turning points—tests of staying power and fortitude. Those bumps in the road can be large or small. They may come and go quickly, or linger and stay awhile. Love from God persists and demonstrates the right way to get through those jolts. Through it all, when we listen and learn, God is good.

Yet, if this is so, why does God allow larger tests of endurance, like suffering and the fight for survival? What purposes do horrific events serve—diseases, sicknesses, floods, and fires? Why are genuinely good people called to bear dismal circumstances? Is God good?

Life is filled with joy alongside sorrow, as God did not promise us a life without distress. He desires instead to grow us. Our development however, does not occur while enjoying top-of-the-peak, excitingly fine times. We develop as we walk trenches enduring trials, much like the vegetation growth that occurs in the valleys. Not much if anything grows on the top of mountains. Humility guides us to accept the path of suffering and develop the stamina required to weather valleys in life, giving wings to endure the mountain climb. Aside from building character, perseverance through valleys permits us to appreciate the breathtaking view from the peak. And what a view it turns out to be.

Can you develop the staying power and fortitude necessary to walk valleys? Climb mountains? Look forward to better times as you endure trials—they are the start of things much greater.

"I hold it true, whate'er befall; I feel it, when I sorrow most;
'Tis better to have loved and lost, than never to have loved at all."
"Love is the only gold."
Alfred, Lord Tennyson

Week Five, Thursday

Individuality

"Teach me your way, O Lord, and I will walk in your truth; give me an undivided heart, that I may fear your name."
Psalm 86:11

Thank heavens for you. With your unique abilities you can uphold solid virtues and see causes through to the end. Stand by your passion. Stay loyal to it and focused on it with conviction. Have courage enough to pursue that desire which has burned for so long in your heart, in the face of seeming forces of opposition.

Celebrate who you are! No other person in this world is exactly like you. Place your best self forward. Strive for improvement, so that God smiles at you, pleased with the "fruit" you are producing: love, joy, peace, patience, kindness, goodness, faithfulness, gentleness, and self-control (Galatians 5:22-23.)

To each individual is given a gift: the day, filled with unique experiences and interactions that add to personality. Cherish those twenty-four hours, using your time wisely to make sure you live each moment and treasure every person who fills your moments. Get to know them with anticipation, like an event you have been looking forward to or a present you are eager to open.

Strengthen your identity in and with every season. Make your mark. Experience fully. You are a person of God's unique creation. Ask yourself what areas of your life call for growth then chart these daily steps toward progress and toward your bequest to society in this lifetime.

"Me. I am me, no one else but me. I think my own thoughts, hope my own hopes, dream my own dreams; No one else is quite the same. That is why I can say: thank you, God, for me."
Me, Australian prayer

Week Five, Friday

Responsible Freedom

"I will walk about in freedom, for I have sought out your precepts."
Psalm 119:45

I miss the playground. Now that my children are older I find my seat is in the car shuttling, rather than in the swing, swinging. Playgrounds represent freedom. We can romp, leap, bounce, and most certainly, swing. Yet they also signify responsibility. When we are old enough we can climb to the highest point in the tower, tackle the monkey bars solo, and careen over beams without hand-holding. This dramatic play in many ways prepares a youngster for life.

Similarly, when we learn how to apply and then use the word of God, responsible freedom characterizes us. We are free to make choices, knowing that the wrong ones yield negative consequences. But when we approach life with good intentions that are matched equally with good actions, we usually enjoy positive outcomes. We play to release pressure and free our spirit. Play balances our working life.

Keep it simple and see what God has in store for you. When was the last time you enjoyed one of life's uncomplicated pleasures, like swinging in a swing? Do you set aside one day each week for rest and play? Are you often too caught up in your work to indulge in play, or perhaps you work at play? Do you play at work? How can you incorporate the enjoyment of God's undemanding pleasures in your life?

"Keeping in touch with childhood memories keeps us believing in life's simplest
pleasures like a rainy afternoon, a swing set, and a giant puddle to play in."
Chrissy Ogden Marsh

Week Five, Saturday

Bondage in Jealousy

"Who is wise and understanding among you? Let them show it by their good life, by deeds done in the humility that comes from wisdom. But if you harbor bitter envy and selfish ambition in your hearts, do not boast about it or deny the truth. Such "wisdom" does not come down from heaven but is earthly, unspiritual, and demonic. For where you have envy and selfish ambition, there you find disorder and every evil practice."
James 3:13-16

Jealousy that stems from self-centered objectives and overzealous protectiveness rapidly twists goodness into distrust and bitterness. Jealousy destroys relationships just as envy and harbored resentment undermine a loving spirit and close off the heart. We can easily fall prey to jealousy's grip when we are not content with who we are, where we are, whom we are with, and when we believe our worth resides in others rather than in God.

Genuine motives and objectives, and an altruistic focus establish an untainted view of special people in our world and free a covetous heart. Safeguard against envy and divert suspicious thinking. Release overprotection and build greater confidence in Elohim, our trustworthy God. Trust permits release from jealousy's stronghold. Since love and suspicion cannot coexist, an envious heart has no room for love, no room for growth. Love thrives with trust and freedom, every month of every season.

When have you felt jealousy try to take you in? Did you yield or steer clear of the temptation? When has envy grown into resentment? What is your defense against jealousy?

"Jealousy comes from self-love rather than from true love."
François VI, Duc de La Rochefoucauld

Week Five, Sunday

Maximize Others, Minimize Self

"Do not boast about tomorrow, for you do not know what a day may bring forth. Let another praise you, and not your own mouth; someone else, and not your own lips."
Proverbs 27:1-2

It's not about you, or your things. Rarely do others care what you require, desire, or acquire. What others will remember is how you focused on them and listened attentively to accounts of priceless details in their lives.

When we drop the self-importance and take on a low profile, less prideful, more modest nature, we experience fulfillment. Think and reflect before words are uttered. Allow thought and reflection to serve as the precursor to action that please others, you, and foremost, your Maker.

A true definition of the word *pride* is often vague and misunderstood. In a positive context, as in "I am proud of you," pride connotes a different meaning than the boastful, vain, arrogant approach to life, often the need to be right, and a source of separation. Void of close ties then, we are unable to raise up others since we are too busy boosting up ourselves. If we lift up only ourselves, chances are we will eventually feel down and then fall down. Rather than boast we can instead boost others. Obtain your own natural elevation and "one-up" someone else with sincere praise. Praise is pure power. Admiration empowers.

How can you minimize *self* and maximize *others*? Can you humble yourself in circumstances that may tempt you to boast, like when you are asked about accomplishments or awards? Can you alter your focus this season to enduringly give your Creator the truly deserved bona fide credit?

"Be a light unto others, not boastful of self."
Edgar Cayce

Freshen Up

This Week

How God leads me . . .

_____
_____
_____
_____
_____
_____
_____

How I follow Jesus . . .

_____
_____
_____
_____
_____
_____
_____

How I hear the Holy Spirit . . .

_____
_____
_____
_____
_____
_____
_____

WEEK SIX

Celebrate Passion

A time to mourn

and

A time to dance

Week Six, Monday

Arrogance Rejects and Separates

"Thus says the Lord: Do not let the wise boast in their wisdom, do not let the mighty let those who boast boast in this, that they understand and know me, that I am the Lord; I act with steadfast love, justice, and righteousness in the earth, for in these things I boast in their might, do not let the wealthy boast in their wealth; but delight, says the Lord."
Jeremiah 9:23-24

Arrogance separates us from God. Egoism considers self to be *all that* in God's eyes, directly deviated from humility. The arrogant self whispers that it is important to look good at another's expense, transmit a sense of false security, and not enlighten others with gifts God has bestowed. Arrogance rejects the wisdom of God and insists on its own way. James 4:16 confirms for us, "As it is, you boast in your arrogance. All such boasting is evil."

Perhaps your desires are to shed ego in order to align with our Creator's overall purpose. Perhaps we recognize arrogance in others, unaware that we have work to do in this area as well. Our relations draw closer to us when we drop the supercilious attitude. Listening to others rather than continual self-direction sends a message that says *I appreciate you* and *friendship with you is a privilege*. We become an approachable, modest friend and even a valued mentor.

When have you let ego get in the way of the real purpose? Can you see relationships in your life as reciprocal interest-interactions? Can you move from me-centered living to a greater you-focused existence? What does *yielding* look like? Are you trying to fit in to your Creator's plan or is it the other way around?

"If America is too arrogant, too prideful to repent, it's not the kind of country that God wants it to be."
Tony Campolo

Week Six, Tuesday

Heartfelt Connections

"For God did not call us to be impure, but to live a holy life. Therefore anyone who rejects this instruction does not reject a human being but God, who gives his holy spirit to you."
1 Thessalonians 4:7-8

Boorish behavior gets uncomfortable. Truthfully, however, most of us exhibit impoliteness from time to time. Rude comments often stem from difficult situations, like when we weather winter seasons in our lives—depleted emotionally, financially, physically—or we become heartbroken and anxious. The list of stressors is endless and can cause us to speak or act out of thoughtless emotion that offends precious people in our circle.

You had a bad day and you need to let off steam. Or perhaps someone was disrespectful or impolite toward you. Give yourself the gift of time to think. Does returning rudeness defray the anger that preceded the offensive behavior or fuel it? Your honest words can be the type of reply you'd like to receive yourself. Then, regardless of the reaction, forgive from the heart. To be certain you won't be one of those rude people everyone runs into from time to time, consistently try to be earnest in your actions to put you and the other person on the same playing field. Heartfelt connections just work.

Rather than confront regrets later, can you find productive ways to channel your pent-up energies like a walk, talk, or leisure time with a friend or pet? Can you take a few moments to consider your response before reacting? Can you pause to ask yourself, *would I want to be treated or spoken to this way?*

"If you wish to be brothers, let the arms fall from your hands. One cannot love while holding offensive arms."
Pope Paul VI

Week Six, Wednesday

Selfless Loyalty

"They would not be like their forefathers—a stubborn and rebellious generation, whose hearts were not loyal to God, whose spirits were not faithful to him."
Psalm 78:8

We cut off possibilities when we insist on our way. We forfeit teachable moments. We fail to see the Master's entrance. Oftentimes we think we know what is best for us, despite repeated disastrous results. Paradoxically, on icy roads I notice that I grip the steering wheel tighter and apply greater pressure to the brakes. Maybe this gives me a false sense of security. Rather than ease up on the brake pedal, the gas, and my grip, allowing for the tires to correct themselves, I attempt to prevent a possible skid with the slam and clench technique. I lose control if the tires lose traction and I grip and force. The same presents itself in daily life: grasp too tight and I may actually lose control. Or I can go along for the ride and enjoy the view out the window, as the learner, taking it all in.

Our all-encompassing, selfless God revealed himself to us by becoming human, as Jesus Christ, and dying for our shortcomings. Without Christ, life is selfish and lonely. We cannot have inner peace without Christ the Redeemer. Our restless hearts vow their own ways, neglecting the goodness gained in relationship with Him. Draw near to Jesus and He draws closer to you.

Have you slipped into the *having it my way* lane on the highway? Do you persist on your path, resistant to teachable moments? Who is truly in control? When have you missed out on intended circumstances or positive personal interaction because you gripped too tight? When were you able to enjoy the view and learn?

"When the pupil is ready, the master will appear."
Ancient proverb

Week Six, Thursday

Blue Nail Polish Eye Shadow

"Satisfy us in the morning with your unfailing love,
that we may sing for joy and be glad all our days."
Psalm 90:14

One day when my youngest daughter was a toddler, she presented me with a nugget of information while I manicured her nails. *"You can learn a lot of lessons from nail polish,"* she announced matter-of-factly. She then presented trivia about how to put on polish with care, especially when using the color blue, adding, *"and you should never put it on your eyelids for eye shadow."* I may have become undone had I witnessed this, but instead I chuckled, knowing this was probably the edifying portion of her inspirational journey. No nail polish on her eyelids that I could see. What I appreciated instead was the enjoyment we had when we were together, perpetually wishing those moments could last longer.

If we get aggravated we lose a sense of fun. How easy for us to grow more agitated as we get older, rather than more patient or playful. How many times have you allowed irritability to take over? What situations provoke even mild annoyances? Why do we let them get the best of us?

Like the blue nail polish eye shadow, can you see the humorous side to details and employ laughter rather than irritation? Next time you get touchy, think about this: is it the other person's behavior or your reaction to the situation that causes irritation? See the circumstances in a different way. See it through their eyes.

"Age does not protect you from love. But love, to some extent, protects you from age."
Jeanne Moreau

Week Six, Friday

Oblivious to Bitterness

"And the Lord's servant must not quarrel; instead, he must be kind to everyone,
able to teach, not resentful."
2 Timothy 2:24

My friend, Maddi, who has Down syndrome, can slide through the same tunnel a dozen times with an unending gigantic grin and loads of giggles. She has a zest and passion for life that most of us lack. I take offense however, at thoughtless, impolite remarks or gestures directed at Maddi, just as if they were directed at me. They make my heart ache, as *I* am equally slighted by these comments.

But I learn from Maddi. She doesn't get offended; she doesn't know bitterness. Maddi is even more precious in God's eyes than any one of us, because she serves as a reminder of how we can look at life clearly, not jaded. She sees each moment as it ought to be seen ~ new, fresh, and fun.

No good comes from harbored anger, since sooner or later bottled-up bitterness surfaces. When it does, there is soon remorse for words or actions. Here is where we can remember a simple three-word phrase: *let it go.*

Bitterness and anger stifle relations, and cause us to look for ways to ease the hurt of a painful memory or event. Investigate the causes of your bitterness or resentment. Write down your thoughts as soon as negative emotions flood in to your being. Find ways to channel your negative energy: walk or talk with a friend, write a letter, verse, or poem, sing, gaze at nature. Recycle offensive behavior into positive, encouraging thoughts and actions. Unload your thoughts in the spirit of prayer to remind you of a more loving attitude and heart. Can you see how working through resentment will allow you to move forward to love more completely? What does that first step look like?

"The only thing we never get enough of is love;
and the only thing we never give enough of is love."
Henry Miller

Week Six, Saturday

Darkness and Light Cannot Coexist

"And out of the ground the Lord God made to grow . . . the tree of knowledge of good and evil. . . For God knows that when you eat of it your eyes will be opened, and you will be like God, knowing good and evil."
Genesis 2:9; 3:5

Most movies draw on a good versus evil theme. Movies can mirror real life: bright vs. ominous; beautiful vs. ugly. Each day we experience tug-of-war, yin-yang trials. Do we choose light or dark? Good or evil? Thoughts and decisions reflect an inner and outer character—an internal struggle to remain steadfast in our belief, and an external conflict between God and Satan. The next time you feel unhappy with a choice, investigate which prompting you followed when you made the decision which eradicated your peace. Those forks in the road are pivotal moments in *your* history.

1 John 1:5-7 reminds us to walk in the light: "This is the message we have heard from him and declare to you: God is light; in him there is no darkness at all. If we claim to have fellowship with him yet walk in the darkness, we lie and do not live by the truth. But if we walk in the light, as he is in the light, we have fellowship with one another, and the blood of Jesus, his Son, purifies us from all sin."

The world bombards us with advertisers who constantly appeal to our desire for high quality, pure, and natural products and methods. We want great not just good—first-class, superior, top-rated stuff. Since many around us say or do things a same certain way, it appears acceptable, even if it clashes with our Creator's plan. So we buy it, do it, or try it. Yet if we strive for pureness in heart we will not tolerate internal or external evil. Darkness and light cannot coexist, so we are not truly living if we endure evil.

How do you discern good from bad? Which paths will you consistently follow? How can you continue to shine intensely amidst dark episodes? Can you grow with a pure heart?

"There are dark shadows on the earth, but its lights are stronger in the contrast."
Charles Dickens

Week Six, Sunday

The Truth Sets Us Free

Jesus answered, "I am the way and the truth and the life. No one comes to the Father except through me. If you really knew me, you would know my Father as well. From now on, you do know him and have seen him."
John 14:6-7

Feelings of betrayal rush through my body as I slouch on the front stoop, sore head in clammy palms one more time. Suffering through an affair and strings of broken promises leave me empty, confused, afraid. Where to turn in this rage-suppressed state? Who to confide in when the comfort rug pulls away? Nothing makes sense any longer, when the entrusted one vanishes, commitments shunned. I am the credulous garment hung to dry. I believed those scandalous lies, time and time again.

When betrayal, the antithesis of truth, or self-serving motives and justifications replace honesty, damage to relationships and separations ensue. The pain of dishonesty pierces our hearts, leaving an open gash. Screaming inside, we question whether we will heal and why we would ever trust or love another once more. Perhaps we've convinced ourselves that little, white lies, withheld information, or false thoughts don't count. Given time we hold onto hope, and, the truth surfaces. Given time we desire an honest life and strong relationships.

We find truth, the real Truth, in God's unmistakable Word, where we are set free and covered in God's loving peace. He knows that nothing can separate us from those we love when strong relations evolve from, flourish in, and remain grounded in His certainty. The Truth brings us closer to God and others. The honesty we gain through Scripture always feels as comfortable as an old, favorite pair of shoes. The Truth sets us free.

Who are you? If you have been challenged with truth-telling even slightly, how can you live in truth despite difficult, tug-of-war situations? Do you speak the truth in love?

"The fastest way to lose our character is to lose our honesty."
Aesop

Celebrate Passion

This Week

How God leads me . . .

_____
_____
_____
_____
_____
_____
_____

How I follow Jesus . . .

_____
_____
_____
_____
_____
_____
_____

How I hear the Holy Spirit . . .

_____
_____
_____
_____
_____
_____
_____

WEEK SEVEN

Thought,

Word,

Deed

A time to scatter stones

and

A time to gather them

Week Seven, Monday

Patience, the Age-Old Talent

"Therefore, as God's chosen people, holy and dearly loved, clothe yourselves
with compassion, kindness, humility, gentleness, and patience."
Colossians 3:12

Patience is not a New Age phenomenon. The poet Ovid enlightened us on this topic over two thousand years ago. Although Ovid didn't wait in a coffee shop line for his double mocha latte, he did realize that patience tests stamina and staying power and that all arrives in its time.

We spend a great deal of our lives waiting. We wait in traffic, we wait in checkout lines, we wait for checks to arrive, and, we wait for answers. The act of hanging in there, whether for an hour, a year, a decade, or much longer requires that we recalibrate our viewpoint to one that feeds patience.

When challenges try patience, refinement has an opportunity to chisel away at our souls. Waiting tests resilience for many of us who want things to work out on our time schedule and we become frustrated when they don't. Tests strengthen patience. Patience builds composure. Then, when composed we find the place of quiet contemplation, turning inward, channeling upward, asking God to guide our thoughts, words, and deeds. Patience allows for true answers rather than the ones we rush into, only to regret later. Events arrive at their appointed times, and not on our clock. There truly is a time for everything and nothing will show up too late.

From love comes a myriad of blessings. Patience is one of those gifts. Was your patience recently tested? How did you stay serene and composed? How can you shift your perspective to maintain patience when necessary?

"Everything comes gradually and at its appointed hour."
Ovid

Week Seven, Tuesday

Power of Touch

"And this is my prayer: that your love may abound more and more
in knowledge and depth of insight."
Philippians 1:9

Love necessitates healthy margins that keep negativity away and retain goodness. There is no capacity-limit to love when real love exists. Deep love opens your heart to unblock your vision and impart a broad reach.

Genuine, limitless love delights in acts of service, protection, encouragement, and more, so much more. Visit an orphanage in a foreign country, and you will experience the pain and loneliness that resides in social orphans. Many orphaned infants and toddlers have never felt warm, human touch, taken refuge in a hug, or known the peace that accompanies a lullaby. Those who serve in orphanages create larger love margins, with the selfless, abounding love and touch they give to orphans who have most likely never known unconditional, bottomless love.

See beyond what presents in the forefront. How can you contribute to the world's needs with abounding love? Can you offer an orphan, a widow, or a shut-in comfort and hope with whole love that accepts the uniqueness of individuals and circumstances? Your world opens up when you unlock another's circumstances.

"Love feels no burden, regards not labors, strives toward more than it attains,
argues not of impossibility, since it believes that it may and can do all things.
Therefore it avails for all things, and fulfills and accomplishes much."
Thomas á Kempis

Week Seven, Wednesday

Dodge Gossip

"Gossips betray a confidence, but the trustworthy keep a secret."
Proverbs 11:13

Rumors. Gossip. Chit chat. He said, she said. There's no harm in a little hearsay, right? After all, it's just a quick story that passes from my lips to someone's ears and nothing more. Besides, the desire burns within to be the first to blurt it out.

Would we feel offended if people held an ambiguous conversation about us while we were not present? If so, then why would we gossip? While gossips may eventually figure out how spiteful words sting, they don't always realize that the tongue is a powerful weapon and cuts as sharp as a sword. Gossip wounds with hurts that often take an extensive time to heal, and frequently cuts deep enough to in no way patch up properly.

Redemption reconciles. Deliverance liberates. We can strive to keep this oath: let me speak solely praiseworthy comments about another person with words the individual would deem acceptable; words that boost their confidence and deepen mutual trust; expressions that bond and bind not sear and scorch. Allow me to spread good words and to be known this way. Let me speak self-assured, as if the other person were directly beside me. My tongue echoes like a powerful instrument, exalted as an uplifting trumpet, with praise and admiration.

When uninvited rumors reach your ears, do you stop the cycle? When have you been a regretful gossip? What were the motivations? Have you asked for forgiveness and made amends, then ceased to gossip? Can you befriend others who also utter only good words?

"What you don't see with your eyes, don't witness with your mouth."
Ancient proverb

Week Seven, Thursday

Discernment

"... preserve sound judgment and discernment, do not let them out of your sight; they will be life for you, an ornament to grace your neck."
Proverbs 3:21-22

Discernment calls us to a higher, more sensitive level in thought, word, and deed. In order to recognize the better outcome, know right from wrong, remain steadfast as a good decision-maker, and above all, to spiritually discriminate the way of life God intends for us from all else the world imposes, we come to value the Spiritual gift of proper judgment. We are challenged to be wise and intelligible in our decision-making, taking into account consequences of our actions and the persons, places, and things involved. When we yearn to discern we unlock our desire to learn. We alter our position. Consequently we yield to development through each season.

A friend and I consulted with each other on the subject of teen children in the house. *These are impressionable years,* we both agreed, realizing that this delicate and sometimes tumultuous span between thirteen and nineteen years of age comes only once per child. During this impressionable period, yet meager time together, our concerns and prayers may be frequent and our advice giving never-ending. We have opportunities to impact the lives of our youth to explain, lead, and mentor them about launching their direction in adulthood and making good choices with proper discernment. Allow God's Spirit to guide during these times. Be familiar with the hallmarks of His authentic nature. Surrender to the overall plan of our Living Stone.

Do you pray prior to decision-making? Do you yield to the Spirit for discernment as you converse with your family, friends, colleagues, or visitors? Have you exercised discernment in formulating decisions that impact other lives and the future? Have you requested discernment from our Teacher?

"We should not fret for what is past, nor should we be anxious about the future; men of discernment deal only with the present moment."
Chanakya

Week Seven, Friday

Never Give Up

"And we know that in all things God works for the good of those who love him,
who have been called according to his purpose."
Romans 8:28

Words from Winston Churchill's speech to the boys at Harrow School in 1941 ring in my ears when I encounter roadblocks. A shorter version of this Churchill quote is etched on a plaque that sits on a shelf in my library. It reads, *Never, never, never give up!* It speaks to me especially on days when I feel challenges surround me; when throwing in the towel and heading back to my comfort chair appears to be the uncomplicated route and clearly the best alternative.

Yet, every day ushers in obstacles. Giving up is an easy option. The right choices are usually a bit tougher and sometimes make us suffer, but in those times we are called to a higher level of personal growth and significant spiritual gain. So under any and all circumstances, never give up, but do remain open to new instructions. Recognize rewards greater than those that are instantly received.

When have you been challenged to never give up? Did you yield to or resist outside forces that attempted to block you from getting where you knew you needed to go? Who in your life has demonstrated that they won't give up—on you, your goals, shared objectives, overall purpose? What loyal persons and virtuous strategies empower you to never give up? Were you willing to ask for and allow help?

"Never, never, in nothing great or small, large or petty, never give in except to
convictions of honour and good sense. Never yield to force; never yield to the
apparently overwhelming might of the enemy."
Sir Winston S. Churchill

Week Seven, Saturday

Global Perspective

Then the Lord said: "I am making a covenant with you. Before all your people I will do wonders never before done in any nation in all the world.
The people you live among will see how awesome is the work
that I, the Lord, will do for you."
Exodus 34:10

In this fast-paced, possession-accumulating world, many families have unconsciously detached from the important issues in life. Perhaps they have merely disengaged from the myriad elements we were all meant to experience and enjoy. Rather than wealth or worldly pleasures, subjects like honesty and wisdom, character and trust, grace and abundance, are central to our development and growth.

As life expectancy increases and converges for most of the world, we live through extended life spans and five co-existing generations who strive to live longer, healthier, wealthier, wiser lives. Despite this mantra, varied age groups voice feeling trapped inside an on-demand, rapid pace era, where society has simply lost focus on life intent, true relations, and gratitude for daily gifts. In spite of having it all people are still discontented, feel empty, search, and continually seek happiness and fulfillment—often in the wrong places.

Does any of this resonate with you? Where do you fit in with today's global perspective? If you strive to break out of the mold, how do you plan to change? Is Christ at the center of your life to provide you with unvarying fulfillment?

"I believe in cultivating opposite, but complementary views of life, and I believe
in meeting life's challenges with contradictory strategies. I believe in reckoning
with the ultimate meaninglessness of our existence, even as we fall in love with
the miracle of being alive. I believe in working passionately to make our lives
count while never losing sight of our insignificance. I believe in caring deeply
and being beyond caring. It is by encompassing these opposites, by being
involved and vulnerable, but simultaneously transcendent and detached,
that our lives are graced by resilience and joy."
Fritz Williams

Week Seven, Sunday

Personal Perspective

"But godliness with contentment is great gain. For we brought nothing into the world, and we can take nothing out of it."
1 Timothy 6:6-7

As long as we keep searching, the answers arrive—for the right solutions, we trust. When we ask ourselves *why* we probe acutely into our main motives—*why* do we do what we do? In the process then, we dive deeper into our reasoning, habits, and unconscious beliefs, ultimately seeking intent. Once we perceive our core motives, we can resolve to change them or to grow them stronger. By regularly asking ourselves *why am I* . . . and *why do I* . . . in a healthy way, we listen closer for the answers that surface in mind, body, and spirit, to produce pure hearts.

In the process, too, we gain a semblance of why, when, and how life plays out. We grasp that in moving through life's problems and possibilities, we discover encounters of both kinds—the seemingly ordinary and the shockingly extraordinary—have purpose in our lives. We value remaining fruitful, modest, and grateful for life's work.

With eyes fixated on Christ, we walk closer to Him and further along in our faith walk. We add depth and breadth to our experiences while strengthening our conviction daily. We learn to lose the temporary in order to gain the eternal. We progress. We grow.

Can you embrace necessary changes rather than resist them? Are you focused daily on God's purpose for you in His overall plan? Have you witnessed progress?

"Bunny slippers remind me of who I am. You can't get a swelled head if you wear bunny slippers. You can't lose your sense of perspective and start acting like a star or a rich lady if you keep on wearing bunny slippers. Besides, bunny slippers give me confidence because they're so jaunty. They make a statement; they say, 'Nothing the world does to me can ever get me so far down that I can't be silly and frivolous.' . . ."
Dean Koontz

Thought, Word, Deed

This Week

How God leads me . . .

How I follow Jesus . . .

How I hear the Holy Spirit . . .

WEEK EIGHT

Forgiveness

and

Acceptance

A time to be embrace

and

A time to refrain

Week Eight, Monday

Defend What is Right

"But let all who take refuge in you be glad; let them ever sing for joy. Spread your protection over them that those who love your name may rejoice in you."
Psalm 5:11

A lioness vigorously protects her cubs for years inside the pride, where adult females safeguard access and defend their cubs from male predators. Male lions patrol their territory boundaries to caution off intruders and maintain ownership of their pride for as long as possible.

Protection, even in the animal kingdom, utilizes its navigation tools, wisdom and discernment, to guard against evil forces that creep in to destroy relationships, undermine individuals, and split families. Love guards and prepares a safe path, yet allows suitable freedom for healthy limits. Love is a shield that defends the just, fair, and right. We lovingly protect when we respect someone's need to be alone during difficult times or to be in company at other times. Love is the protector. Defend love; look after it. Love is our greatest gift.

If you are fortunate enough to have loved ones who support, defend, and visit at two in the morning when you call on them, you are truly blessed. If this is the type of companionship we desire, certainly it is the friendship we give and defend.

Do we stifle love when we overprotect, albeit with good intentions, but only to end up creating insecurity? When have you set love free rather than cocoon it and allowed God to protect love? Were you able to discern proper thoughts and actions to make the right decisions? How can you build a fortress of protection for healthy, loving relationships? What about for your community or network? What about for the world? God the Protector sees us through all circumstances.

"Lots of people will want to ride with you in the limo, but what you want is someone who will take the bus with you when the limo breaks down."
Oprah Winfrey

Week Eight, Tuesday

Hope All Things

But as for me, I will always have hope; I will praise you more and more."
Psalm 71:14

Hope can propel us into the next day when life presents hurdles directly where we stand. With hope and unyielding trust in God's will we can once more look forward to the future, desire effective changes, and anticipate progress. Hope is all some people profess to go on from day to day.

Extreme weather events present uncontrollable scenarios. Natural disasters do not discriminate, as they equalize rich and poor, black and white. Hardships set ruin into people's homes and hearts. The 2004 Indian Ocean earthquake and tsunami took the lives of 230,000 people in fourteen countries. Hurricane Katrina of 2005, one of the deadliest in nearly eighty years, displaced the general population of Mississippi and Louisiana for over five years. The 2008 storm surge that inundated Burma created widespread damage that also affected the world. In these and numerous similar situations, people searched for loved ones, remainders of their homes, and belongings for years. Most were left with nothing.

Nothing but hope that is. Devastating events however, have had a way of inciting wide-range humanitarian reactions that infuse hope and love and are connected by faith rather than dissuaded by fear. This combination—hope, love, and faith—shifts people into action. As we search for love, we hope to find it and do when we are faithful to our overall purpose first. Once we place conditions on love, we lose faith, and eventually, hope. Hope flourishes when free and encouraged, while in the presence of love. As 1 Corinthians 13:13 reminds us, "Three things will last forever—faith, hope, and love—and the greatest of these is love."

What is your outlook on hope? Despite experiences of unrealized hopes, can you sustain an optimistic view? How do you get up and go on after defeat? When has love enhanced hope? Do you lean on the Rock, God Almighty, who supplies hope every day?

"We are all in the gutter, but some of us are looking at the stars. What seems to us as bitter trials are often blessings in disguise."
Oscar Wilde

Week Eight, Wednesday

Accept That You Are Adequate

"I have loved you with an everlasting love. I have drawn you with loving-kindness."
Jeremiah 31:3

If I'm alright and you're alright, then why do I feel this way? Have you ever experienced this sensation? Superficially, a lack of self-acceptance provides the rationale for a person's lack of confidence to bind them to healthy external relations. But what resides at the core?

God loves and accepts us right where we are today. Many people, even Christians, have an arduous time grasping that God doesn't demand perfection; he merely requests obedience so that he can draw us in closer. Just to know and experience God's uncompromising and accepting love ought to grant us sufficient understanding, warmth, and acceptance to transmit to others.

We were created with uncompromised love and are provided constant reminders. Created in His image, we were set free. We can grow to love and accept ourselves and others including the built-in flaws, without qualifiers, *regardless* of whether others accept or reject us. God's everlasting love surpasses any provisions. God's word provides us with the foundation for wholesome interpersonal relationships and affirms that He accepts us just as we are, right where we are. Herein remains the foundation of faith.

Do you think well of yourself or do you feel the need to please others in order to be accepted? What stirs up thoughts or feelings of inadequacy? Has rejection caused you to pull away from relationships? Have you sought approval from others in place of fulfilled desires, passions, or goals, or a closer relationship with God? God meets us where we are and accepts us as we are.

"If I know what love is, it is because of you. Some of us think that holding on makes us strong; but sometimes it is letting go."
Herman Hesse

Forgiveness and Acceptance

Week Eight, Thursday

It's Not Too Late

Peter replied, "Repent and be baptized, every one of you, in the name of Jesus Christ for the forgiveness of your sins. And you will receive
the gift of the Holy Spirit."
Acts 2:38

Years ago a friend from work spoke to Kyle repeatedly about forgiveness. Kyle had sought a church every so often but never followed through. First he merely walked by the church when the doors were open during services. Eventually he walked up the steps of this church and listened from the entrance, then the vestibule, then the back row of seats.

Now, after fourteen years, a failed marriage, two children, and yet another job loss, Kyle was finally starting to "get it." He confessed his sins. God listened as Kyle renounced his life to Him with prayers and sobs. God heard Kyle's pleas for forgiveness for his many shortcomings as well as his gratitude for many blessings, so richly sprinkled on him throughout his life. *Even now.* Never before had Kyle felt such a weight lifted from him. He felt free.

Growing in faith has been a continual process for Kyle, who still struggles daily with control versus relinquishment during his tumultuous days. Surrender with trust became the focal point for Kyle then and remains so today. His battles gave him freedom to fully accept his Heavenly Father's forgiveness, walking through life in the path He sets before him.

Do you know these kinds of struggles? Have you fully given in to accept forgiveness? It's never too late to grow closer to Christ, and to strive for a Christ-like life. Receive deliverance by reading and accepting *The Prayer* in the Closing Moments. Christ Jesus awaits you.

"God grant me the serenity to accept the things I cannot change, the courage to change the things I can, and the wisdom to know the difference."
Reinhold Niebuhr

Week Eight, Friday

Guilt-free Living

"I will cleanse them from all the guilt of their sin against me, and I will forgive all the guilt of their sin and rebellion against me."
Jeremiah 33:8

A friend found herself in a sticky situation with another friend who asked that she not repeat a story. After all, it involved someone dear to both of them. Upon coercion she spilled the beans anyway. Shame, guilt, and betrayed trust entered the former long-term bond for all three friends.

Guilt leaves us with an empty feeling inside. We feel remorseful once we've wronged someone and resentment when we find ourselves on the other side of the fence. After our wrongful acts, forgiveness directed first at ourselves helps us make amends with the other person later. As grueling as forgiveness is for some people it is necessary in order to reposition the relationship. Avoid nagging thoughts and sleepless nights: Forgive.

Blame and fault-finding provide roots for guilt. Have you felt self-reproach, even trepidation, over a matter in which you ought to have felt innocence? What provoked these guilt feelings—was it fear, a surplus of responsibility, or a lack of accountability for your decisions or actions? Was it a feeling of separation from the Source? What roused feelings of guilt for something that occurred in your past? How did you release the guilt? Can you help create guilt-free days for you and significant others in your life? Can you live without criticism, regret, or blame? Father God sent his son Jesus Christ to forgive all those who believe. Forgiveness is one of the greatest gifts our Redeemer gave to us.

"Every man is guilty of all the good he didn't do."
Voltaire

Week Eight, Saturday

Forgive to Make it Right

"Instead, be kind and tender-hearted to one another, and forgive one another,
as God forgave you through Christ."
Ephesians 4:32

You may never get an apology. Then what? Remaining stuck in resentment is not a healthy option. Forgiveness is a process that takes healing from the inside, out. Healing takes place once you acknowledge the hurt and forgive yourself or the offender. Make the important decision to forgive an offense whether it is the first, seventh, or seventy times seventh time—seek atonement and let go. Our spirits become squelched when we don't show mercy, get beyond the hurt, and forgive others and ourselves. Relentless forgiveness, even if merely in your heart, opens the gates to more love, more goodness, and more life.

Hawaiians have a ceremony to facilitate healing called Ho'oponopono, or Pono, meaning *to make right*. They release harbored, negative emotions that create toxins leading to ill health for body, mind, and spirit. They believe that a positive attitude and a non-hostile, anger-free environment are essential to restore balance and sustain optimal health.

Think back on a time when you needed forgiveness. If your apology was accepted, was there restitution? If you were the one offering atonement but it was rejected, have you been able to release any false feelings of guilt and shame? Have you demonstrated mercy, outwardly expressed forgiveness, or forgiven in your heart? How have *you* been able to heal when you've made it right?

"Forgive, forgive, and forgive some more. Never stop forgiving, for the
temptation to project and judge will always be there as long as you are living in
the body. Forgiveness is the key to peace and happiness, and gives us everything
that we could possibly want."
Gerald G. Jampolsky

Week Eight, Sunday

Gifts to One Another

"Then Peter began to speak: 'I now realize how true it is that God does not show favoritism but accepts those from every nation who fear him and does what is right. You know the message God sent to the people of Israel, announcing the good news of peace through Jesus Christ, who is Lord of all.'"
Acts 10:34-36

We are gifts to one another. Why would we show prejudice or a judgmental nature? Negativity and a critical spirit display a narrow-minded outlook and thwart the global objective we were meant to develop. See other individuals for their unique, innate qualities. There is much more to a person than color, culture, or creed. Why let race, age, or religion impede the potential for a great relationship?

The people of this world are diverse, but more alike than essentially recognized. Give applause and a standing ovation for diversity, for without it we would live in a dull, lackluster world. Have a deeper look at an individual's character for unapparent commonalities or attractive differences, rather than skin tone, outer wear, hair or eye color. When we are open to a sundry of healthy relations, we form powerful connections.

Many of us will never know what it is like for persons of a certain race or ethnicity to suffer physical, psychological, or spiritual oppression. How often do you demonstrate objectivity and impartiality? Have you been able to make friends without bias? Are you fair and neutral?

"Our senses don't deceive us: our judgment does."
Johann Wolfgang von Goethe

Forgiveness and Acceptance

This Week

How God leads me . . .

How I follow Jesus . . .

How I hear the Holy Spirit . . .

Summer

Hot and sultry days
Life abounds and envelops us
Lively months ahead

Bathing in the sun
Time for walks, talks, pondering
Gather and reflect

© Gabriella D. Filippi

WEEK NINE

Exalt,

Glorify,

Praise

A time to search

and

A time to give up

Week Nine, Monday

Hum Drum or Drum and Hum?

"Sing to the LORD a new song; sing to the LORD, all the earth."
Psalm 96:1

Melinda, a thirty-four-year-old homemaker, was worn down by the tedious, repetitive nature of each day. Sometimes she changed her morning routine and watched the *AM Live Show*, other droning days Melinda attempted a new recipe.

Then one day Melinda discovered a lump under her armpit. For several days she ignored it, thinking it would disappear. When the scenario didn't change, she went to her doctor. After subsequent appointments, Melinda received life-altering news. A biopsy revealed that the mass was cancerous, and the affected area had expanded. Surgery followed by chemotherapy was her best option but even then there was a thirty percent chance of survival. Melinda's world turned 180 degrees during those next few months, vacillating between life and death.

Although Melinda survived cancer, her attitude changed. To place a wig or hat on her head *one more time* was not so bad anymore, considering that she was still able to hold her three year old *one more time*. Tedious doctor visits were less routine and more gratifying as she visualized everyone's face at the dinner table, together again, *one more time*. What had become transparent now to Melinda was what she had heard countless times before and was altogether true: life passes quickly.

During those mundane moments and ordinary hours we can arrive at epiphanies that alter life. Do we listen with intent, see with clarity, live fully? Our vaporous days in earthly existence are numbered. Do we cease to acknowledge common epiphanies or live one prized moment at a time?

"The secret of happiness is to find a congenial monotony."
Sir Victor Sawdon Pritchett

Week Nine, Tuesday

Hope All Things

"But as for me, I will always have hope; I will praise you more and more."
Psalm 71:14

Hope can propel us into the next day when life presents hurdles directly where we stand. With hope and unyielding trust in God's will we can once more look forward to the future, desire effective changes, and anticipate progress. Hope is all some people profess to go on from day to day.

Extreme weather events present uncontrollable scenarios. Natural disasters do not discriminate, as they equalize rich and poor, black and white. Hardships set ruin into people's homes and hearts. The 2004 Indian Ocean earthquake and tsunami took the lives of 230,000 people in fourteen countries. Hurricane Katrina of 2005, one of the deadliest in nearly eighty years, displaced the general population of Mississippi and Louisiana for over five years. The 2008 storm surge that inundated Burma created widespread damage that also affected the world. In these and numerous similar situations, people searched for loved ones, remainders of their homes, and belongings for years. Most were left with nothing.

Nothing but hope that is. Devastating events however, have had a way of inciting wide-range humanitarian reactions that infuse hope and love and are connected by faith rather than dissuaded by fear. This combination—hope, love, and faith—shifts people into action. As we search for love, we hope to find it and do when we are faithful to our overall purpose first. Once we place conditions on love, we lose faith, and eventually, hope. Hope flourishes when free and encouraged, while in the presence of love. As 1 Corinthians 13:13 reminds us, "Three things will last forever—faith, hope, and love—and the greatest of these is love."

What is your outlook on hope? Despite experiences of unrealized hopes, can you sustain an optimistic view? How do you get up and go on after defeat? When has love enhanced hope? Do you lean on the Rock, God Almighty, who supplies hope every day? Can you praise Him even during the storms?

"We are all in the gutter, but some of us are looking at the stars. What seems to us as bitter trials are often blessings in disguise."
Oscar Wilde

Week Nine, Wednesday
Modern Day Miracle

"You saw with your own eyes the great trials, the miraculous signs and wonders,
the mighty hand and outstretched arm,
with which the Lord your God brought you out."
Deuteronomy 7:19

I phoned mom on a Tuesday evening for some girl talk. Dad had passed away about ten months earlier and she expressed the emotional, physical, and even spiritual weariness from this new life without her companion. I decided to comfort her with Scripture supporting God's protection of widows and orphans.

Early Thursday morning, just two days later, we spoke again.

Well, I'm on the road, she sheepishly replied when I asked what she was doing. She referred to the long travel to monitor construction progress of their retirement home—my father's "last dream"—the vision he never lived to see.

Who's going with you? I inquired, realizing that only my brothers or I have taken this four-hour trek with mom. Perhaps it was the severe rainstorm forecasted for later in the day or the fact that only dad, never mom, had taken this expedition alone, but instant concern swept over me as she responded, I'm *driving alone.* I asked her to phone me on her journey home.

Hours later I received a call from a hospital emergency department. While traveling home, my mother's vehicle rolled three times at sixty five miles per hour, landing on its hood in the median of the highway, contents hurled from inside. Miraculously, no other vehicle or property was involved. She had crawled out of the shattered front windshield, escaping the accident with only minor bruises.

My brother cried in disbelief when he identified mother's automobile with all windows shattered, hood brutally compressed, tire blown, and irreparable body damage. In the State Trooper's words, *we don't see people survive these kinds of crashes.* When I asked mom to describe the sensation that very few live to tell of—rolling in a fast-moving vehicle—she replied, *I felt at peace.*

I believe that God came through in a big way on a rainy, autumn afternoon in 2008. He replaced mom's emotional, physical, and Spiritual stressors that season with His peace. God requires faith and not proof, yet this modern-day miracle confirmed truthful Scripture: Fear nothing. God is our Protector. Our omnipotent Father is a loving God of His word. Praise His glorious name.

Have you seen or felt God's amazing love? Have you witnessed a modern day miracle?

"A father to the fatherless, a defender of widows, is God in his holy dwelling."
Psalm 68:5

Week Nine, Thursday

The Gardener

"I am the vine, and My Father is the vinedresser. Every branch in me that does not bear fruit, He takes away; and every branch that bears fruit, He prunes it, that it may bear more fruit."
John 15:1-2

Karl Forester's feather reed grass is surely a most favorite perennial plant for many. Straw and green plumes ripple sway with the wind and stand at attention when the breeze absconds. Alone the plant stands simply elegant; majestic when clustered in a garden.

The gardener has a mission. She sees her design in her dreams. Her mind creates a vision prior to staking her plot. Planting is a ritual, at which she is the master. Each hole she digs, every bulb, annual, perennial, tree, bush, and flowering plant eased into the ground depends upon her firm, yet gentle, guiding hands. She takes care to delicately prune branches that are no longer alive, and trim back others to become healthier. The gardener exalts His Holy Name as she toils.

The Master Gardener in our lives has planted seeds within us all. One of our inherent purposes is to discern just when, where, and how those plants will grow. He knows what venue best suits our flourishing.

Visualize a colorful bouquet just for you. This bunch contains cheerful moments, represented by flourishing flowers in bloom, and grim times, those characterized by lean, withering ones. What does your collection resemble? Does your garden require planting, pruning, or watering? Have you asked the Gardener to help you bear more fruit?

"If I'm ever reborn, I want to be a gardener—
there's too much to do for one lifetime!"
Karl Foerster

Week Nine, Friday

Be the Thread

"Train up a child in the way he should go, and when he is old,
he will not depart from it."
Proverbs 22: 6

I am not kidding when I say that I miss the kid in my kid. He grew up right before me in moments, not years. I can still hear his tiny voice and giggles, as I would burrow my head into his belly to make us both laugh. When did my sweet little boy walk out the door as an independent young man? Did we share enough lasting memories? Did I maintain an unyielding thread between us?

While I miss that boy in all his innocence and curiosity, I wouldn't miss the seasonal progressions for anything. Is it possible that we lose the kid only to regain it later? If we live right, perhaps we were meant to never stop being childlike—uncomplicated, trusting, pure. Although the physical cord is disconnected at birth, the relational thread ought to grow stronger in time, through love and grace.

Raising children requires patience and time, two essentials ingredients many parents stock in short supply. While children deserve our full attention, by the close of a busy day we may feel as though we are at the end of an unraveling rope, giving them far less than their quota. Kids do love it when we spend time with them. Pastor Phillip Way in Round Rock, Texas revealed an interesting manner to define TIME: *T*ogether for *I*nspiration, *M*otivation, and *E*ncouragement. Doesn't this say it all?

How much T-I-M-E have you spent with the K-I-D in your life today? How do you oversee the mental, physical, and spiritual fibers to his being? Is the thread between your child and you twisted, knotted, perhaps separating, or is it intact, wholesome, and strong? How can you thicken the cord by strengthening the tie?

"Kids spell love T-I-M-E."
John Crudele

"My mom and dad love me no matter what."
Abbey, age 8

Week Nine, Saturday

Rhythm

"Do not conform any longer to the pattern of this world, but be transformed by the renewing of your mind. Then you will be able to test and approve what God's will is—His good, pleasing, and perfect will."

Romans 12:2

Listen to rain. Do you feel the rhythm that you hear? Gentle tapping that is soothing, calming, and inviting. Envisage all life forms peaceful while experiencing warm, quiet, comfortable rainfall. God has surely placed things in ideal order.

Life has a rhythm. There is a cadence that sets each day in motion. Our routines structure a pattern that brings regularity to our days' activities. We follow sequences, progressing according to the habitual order we arrange. Do you like your tempo? Or do you wish to alter the pulse?

Change discordant beats. Keep life in motion. Each day, renew your mind with the Lord. Commence your days with five P's: pure psyche prepared (for) positive progression. Open your thoughts. Release old patterns holding you hostage, so you carry on rooted in a healthy cycle. If you are despondent because of your current pace, create new momentum. Feel the tempo, be the cadence. Modify the way you think and act so that you can shift gears and maintain rhythm. Establish your rhythm of harmony in life so you can then tune in to the cadence of Christ.

"Happiness is not a matter of intensity but of balance, order,
rhythm, and harmony."
Thomas Merton

Week Nine, Sunday

Themes

"Finally, brothers, whatever is true, whatever is noble, whatever is right, whatever is pure, whatever is lovely, whatever is admirable—if anything is excellent or praiseworthy—think about such things."
Philippians 4:8

If you lived to be eighty years old and filled a basket with significant memories from your childhood to adulthood, what items would amass inside? Various themes—belonging, freedom, loss—have shaped the memories in your life—images, experiences, inspirations. How full is your basket? How colorful? Which accounts have impressed upon you most? The following phrases may unlock your thoughts for this exercise:

Meditate. Close your eyes and slow your breathing as you are in the moment, the here and now. Still the mind chatter to invite thoughtful reflection. What senses are heightened? Is your imagination more vivid?

Picture a day that was filled with anticipation. What did that feel like? Did the expectation of an occasion feel more exciting than the actual event?

Saying something special aloud about someone stirs up emotions. List a handful—at least three—positive, uplifting attributes about a friend. How does this make you both feel?

Fill a bag with dreams, each written on a separate piece of paper. These dreams could be ones you have anticipated for years or have presently formulated. Which one do you hope you retrieve first? What is limiting you from fulfilling this dream?

What are your desires for the remaining contents of this theme basket? Rather than altering goals, can you visualize changing your steps to accomplish them? What is more important to you—the quality or the quantity of the contents you place in your basket? How do the contents of your basket reflect God's plans for you?

"I shut my eyes in order to see."
Eugène Henri Paul Gauguin

Exalt, Glorify, Praise

This Week

How God leads me . . .

_____
_____
_____
_____
_____
_____
_____

How I follow Jesus . . .

_____
_____
_____
_____
_____
_____
_____

How I hear the Holy Spirit . . .

_____
_____
_____
_____
_____
_____
_____

WEEK TEN

Give and Receive;

Bless and Be Blessed

A time to keep

and

A time to throw away

Week Ten, Monday

Kindness Blesses Both Giver and Receiver

"Get rid of all bitterness, rage and anger, brawling and slander, along with every form of malice. Be kind and compassionate to one another, forgiving each other, just as in Christ God forgave you."
Ephesians 4:31-32

When friends bless us with genuinely thoughtful words or when we provide that same support, we feel inspired, uplifted, and even renewed, don't we? Kind actions match the volume of kind words. Humanitarian acts require that we take ourselves out of the equation and focus on compassion. Alas when we are kind to others, we are changed. Not only do our acts of kindness change us, they influence others. If everyone displayed a small act of kindness every day, we'd all be in a more comfortable place, now wouldn't we?

Put your heart as well as your head into the situation—place yourself in another person's position. Though you may not have experienced a major life event like the death of a loved one or cancer, consideration toward someone in those circumstances, with kind words and actions, extends further than we conceive. Maybe, just maybe, these situations experienced by people placed in your path foreshadow events yet to transpire in your life, and provide a nudge to show kindness rather than wait for it to come to you.

Reflect on someone who has been attentive and kind, conceivably a benevolent mentor to you. How were you blessed by this individual? When have you acted with sincere kindness in another person's life?

"Kind words do not cost much, yet they accomplish much."
Blaise Pascal

Week Ten, Tuesday

Relational Depth Not Debt

"Dear friends, let us love one another, for love comes from God. Everyone who loves has been born of God and knows God. Whoever does not love does not know God, because God is love."
1 John 4:7-8

Do you know someone with a hardened heart? Perhaps this describes you? As I enter my home any time of day or night, my dogs greet me with wagging tails and wet slobbers. Their body language says *we love you, no matter what*. It brings an instant grin to my face, knowing that without any strings attached, I get to experience unqualified love from my canine friends.

When you think of adding depth to a relationship, what comes to mind? Is absolute, unrestricted, total love an option for humans? Our parents loved us to this depth. And without fail, our Father God loves us beyond measure, without conditions. God is love, and love is and comes from God. If love is God then we know love is supreme. Yet do we place love as our highest standard? No qualifiers, no conditions, just pure love given freely, no matter what. Do you see all people as individuals like you, with the same basic needs that you have? If you wore blinders and could not differentiate skin color, limitations, size, and shape, how might this alter your ability to accept and love people merely for who they are?

Chip away at toughness, beginning with your own lack of sensitivity. To elevate healthy relations in your life, move beyond accustomed limits to give wholehearted love and reach a greater depth in relationships. For those in your life who are difficult to love, what if you were the one who loved first? Are you too conditioned in a committed relationship to maintain spontaneity and instinctual, unrestricted love? Do you place conditions on unconditional love? Close your eyes and visualize open arms that await you at anytime. Are your arms always open?

"Throughout life people will make you mad, disrespect you and treat you bad.
Let God deal with the things they do,
cause hate in your heart will consume you, too."
Will Smith

Week Ten, Wednesday

Live Outside Yourself

"Do nothing from selfishness or conceit, but in humility count others better than yourselves. Let each of you look not only to his own interests, but also to the interests of others. Have this mind among yourselves, which you have in Christ Jesus."
Philippians 2:3-5

Hard work has merit beyond the tasks involved. For instance, ask yourself, are you motivated by the prospect of gaining? Humility places *I* and *me* out of the picture and considers others better than self. Authenticity manifests through selfless living, when our efforts are directed outside of and beyond self. I met a man who spoke of the impact his ski accident had on his life outlook. He valued living more now that he was in a wheelchair, and prized it like a gift thereafter.

He explained how, prior to his accident, he was selfish and self-absorbed in his affluent lifestyle. After he had healed—physically, mentally, emotionally, and spiritually—he avowed that he was better equipped to give and inspire people. He had more now that he *chose* to hoard less. In his words, he was blessed, truly blessed.

When we serve others and live outside of ourselves we bring purpose to our occupancy on earth. Have you experienced past occurrences when you were selfish or self-absorbed in your approach to life or love? How did you feel? How can you begin to incorporate an altruistic attitude and feel exalted?

"The true joy of life is being used for a purpose recognized by yourself as a mighty one . . . being thoroughly worn out before you are thrown to the scrap heap . . . being a force of nature instead of a feverish, selfish clod of ailments and grievances."
George Bernard Shaw

Week Ten, Thursday

Delayed Gratification

> "For the creation was subjected to frustration, not by its own choice, but by the will of the one who subjected it, in hope that the creation itself will be liberated from its bondage to decay and brought into the freedom and glory of the children of God."
> Romans 8:20-21

This very topic of delayed gratification was addressed in a school circular, suggesting that delaying gratification in our children positions them for a more prominent future. If children who postpone pleasures become more successful in life, I wondered, what would this say for adults who choose to model this behavior?

Debt is at its all-time high for today's society. Delaying gratification purely can mean that the will exists to go without for the time being, with the aim of making gains later. Financial freedom draws from the delayed gratification bank with the thought that sacrifices at present yield long-term success. Contrary to certain philosophies, greed is not good. While every dream has a price, it usually requires patience and intuitive timing. If it's meant to be, it will.

Write down your heart's desires for now, and five, ten, and fifteen years from now, keeping them safe yet accessible. Alongside these dreams and desires, formulate a pithy list of temptations that might divert you from the goal by doing something instantly satisfying. Hence, these temptations could take you a few steps back from the goal. Does fulfillment arrive as patience and perseverance grow? Can delayed gratification actually bring greater satisfaction?

> "We live in a prosperous nation, but people have mortgaged their future. Debt is standing in the way of a brighter future . . . People haven't been taught delayed gratification."
> Gregory Petsch

Week Ten, Friday

Gratitude, the Beginning

"In everything give thanks, for this is the will of God."
1 Thessalonians 5:18

Many of us enjoy comfortable lives. Most days lack mind's eye for a "high" point; alas plenty of "lows" can be recited. Why do we focus on the negative? Does it make us feel better to express ourselves in a style of self-pity?

Gratitude releases our senses and alters our mind set, actually calling for mindfulness. There is no faux pas involved in recognizing attitude as part of the word gratitude. We free our spirit, sending our psyche to greater heights when we live in a gratitude mode. Everything appears promising versus pitiful. A constructive, razor-sharp attitude sets everything in motion.

Give thanks. Today, list at least five items that cannot be bought or borrowed, for which you are most grateful. Ponder over them. Then tomorrow list another five and do the same the next day. Continue with this daily regimen until you learn to begin and end each day in gratitude.

> "Gratitude unlocks the fullness of life. It turns what we have into enough, and more. It turns denial into acceptance, chaos into order, confusion into clarity. It can turn a meal into a feast, a house into a home, a stranger into a friend. Gratitude makes sense of our past, brings peace for today, and creates a vision for tomorrow."
> Melody Beattie

Week Ten, Saturday

Gratitude, the Continuum

> "Let the word of Christ dwell in you richly, in all wisdom, teaching and
> admonishing each other, in psalms, and hymns, and spiritual songs,
> in grace singing in your hearts to the Lord."
> Colossians 3:16

So easily we take, not give; receive, but not counter with an offering of our own. Do we overlook small gestures of kindness that speak to our souls in a deep way, yet forgo the opportunity to express gratitude when it presents itself? Begin a gratitude-training program for yourself, by yourself, about yourself initially. Give thanks for all the qualities you possess, talents that inspire you, passions that move you into action. Make this a priority daily.

Secondarily, create acute appreciative awareness for all those in your life who motivate you with their genuine eagerness to learn and grow, who reposition your attention to what truly matters in life. Focus on them, expressing genuine thanks regularly in words and deeds.

Lastly, concentrate on the individuals whose lives you have or will touch, who also inspire you with their authentic fervor to gain knowledge, be taught, and develop. These are people you serve, as you fulfill your highest calling. Openly convey your heartfelt appreciation in thoughts and actions. Begin and end each day in thanks.

> "As we express our gratitude, we must never forget that the highest
> appreciation is not to utter words, but to live by them."
> John F. Kennedy

Week Ten, Sunday

Gratitude, the Finale

"I thank Christ Jesus Our Lord, who has given me strength to do His work. He considered me trustworthy and appointed me to serve Him."
1Timothy 1:12

Have you received enough today to sustain your existence? Has your family's well being been fulfilled? Has the Lord given you this day your daily bread?

Each day we have the opportunity to utter thank you—yet we miss the chance if we feel it but do not say it. Thank you for my baby's gurgles and my child's laughter, right along with their sicknesses and cries. They remind me of what is important in life. Thank you for my husband's gainful employment and the ability to provide for our family. Thank you for my workload that keeps me vested in goals and projects inside and outside the home. Thank you for my parents, who brought me into and involved me in this world. Thank you for my friends who anticipate my needs, as I do theirs. Lord, I desire to serve you with an ever-grateful heart.

Gratitude liberates insight, your pathway to wisdom. How often do you express *thank you* throughout the day? Have you been grateful in your deeds as well as your words? Why do you feel gratitude? Note circumstances and feelings, as they are apt to come about more readily as you recognize moments of gratitude.

"Feeling you are grateful and not expressing it is like wrapping a present and not giving it."
William Arthur Ward

Give and Receive; Bless and Be Blessed

This Week

How God leads me . . .

_____
_____
_____
_____
_____
_____
_____

How I follow Jesus . . .

_____
_____
_____
_____
_____
_____
_____

How I hear the Holy Spirit . . .

_____
_____
_____
_____
_____
_____
_____

WEEK ELEVEN

Broken but Willing;

Reduce and Grow

A time to tear

and

A time to mend

Week Eleven, Monday

Broken

"My grace is sufficient for you, for my power is made perfect in weakness. Therefore I will boast all the more gladly about my weaknesses, so that Christ's power may rest on me. That is why, for Christ's sake, I delight in weaknesses, in insults, in hardships, in persecutions, in difficulties. For when I am weak,
then I am strong."
2 Corinthians 12:9-10

Break me down. Reduce me to rawness. Allow me to see my greatest flaws so that I may quickly strengthen my bleakest weaknesses. For it is when I am broken that I am subservient, willing to learn, and I can build back up even stronger.

We all become broken at some point. Often times it is over and over again. We seek to put together the fragmented, broken pieces of our lives very much as a mosaic would be fashioned, arriving at a beautiful work of art, placed together piece by piece. This simple complexity exists universally. Broken as well at least once or twice, an angel with a broken wing is a divine messenger who comforts the oppressed and oppresses the comfortable. For it is through our brokenness that we become stronger, resisting temptation to martyr, happy with our choices.

Brokenness brings us to our knees. With our selfish options exhausted, we sit teachable, ask for mercy, plead for grace, and search for instant clemency to avoid the inescapable. For it is through God's benevolence that we are clean again.

Break me down. Allow the brokenness in my life to gradually piece together my heart and make enough sense to create a montage of beauty that instills order and harmony in me.

Break me down. Test my heart. Build my spirit. Let the real growing begin in my life.

Break me down. Position me. Grow me again from the inside out.

"Blessed are the hearts that can bend; they shall never be broken."
Albert Camus

Week Eleven, Tuesday

Gold and Silver

"I will shake all nations, and the desired of all nations will come, and I will fill this house with glory,' says the Lord Almighty. 'The silver is mine and the gold is mine,' declares the Lord Almighty. 'The glory of this present house will be greater than the glory of the former house,' says the Lord Almighty. 'And in this place I will grant peace,' declares the Lord Almighty."
Haggai 2:7-9

All that is of value belongs to the Lord God. Both the Haggai verse above and Revelation 20 reference the Messiah and the millennial, a thousand-year time period of holiness during which Jesus and his faithful followers are to rule on earth for a long awaited age of joy, serenity, righteousness, and success. *The wealth or precious things of all nations* refers to the offerings the nations will bring to the millennial temple, which will contain the *glory* and splendor of the Lord's presence. Nations will lay everything at the feet of the Master of the Universe, despite boasting of their riches and prosperity, as the Messiah, the Prince of Peace, will reign in the millennial kingdom.

What does the gold and silver in your life look like? Each of my children learned a familiar song when young, with an emphatic chorus: M*ake new friends, but keep the old; one is silver and the other gold.* New friends and old friends are both gold and silver. Both are valuable, purposeful gifts from God that belong to Him. Both forms of friendship can modify and be rewritten over time, revive, then sustain and mature. Friendships refine like metals. Certainly what is genuine will endure. Friendships that are grounded in Christ's love and season gracefully are the greatest gifts of all in life. However, it is impossible to be a follower and friend of Christ, and also retain the closeness of all friends and neighbors, when the Holy Spirit rests within us. He purifies us and directs our thoughts so that we know in certainty the steps we ought to take on the narrow path before us. The Lord is faithful to those who obediently commit to perform His work for the glory of God.

Who is your best friend? What does your friendship circle look like? Who are the true friends in your *temple*? Are you a kind and genuine friend that is first focused on loyalty to the Lord of hosts? Do you present the Lord with gold and silver each day?

"I can trust my friends. These people force me to examine, encourage me to grow."
Cher

Week Eleven, Wednesday

Hats

"Listen to advice and accept instruction, and in the end you will be wise. Many are the plans in a man's heart, but it is the Lord's purpose that prevails."
Proverbs 19:20-21

We can wear many different hats in this journey. Certainly, we could be in search of just the right one for an entire lifetime. Or, we could try on several during the course of our existence, keeping them on, enjoying them while we wear them, and move on to the next hat when the prompting arrives. Whichever hat(s) we choose while we are searching, how can we make certain we enjoy the wearing of the one intended for us?

While searching for the right hat, exude anticipation and a chance to shift and explore talents and opportunities. What lies on the horizon is for an exciting discovery. Often times however, it is necessary to back up a few steps to gain a running start before fully accelerating forward.

Today is a gift, so open up the present intently, taking note of each moment as it unfolds. Our days are numbered. Seek a time to *be* more, and *do* less—take pleasure in peaceful *being* rather than busy *doing*. Seek and exist with an open mind, body, and spirit. Seek rejuvenation, discoveries, renewal. Whether you call them hats or identify them as goals and ambitions are you sporting the one(s) intended for you by our Master Designer?

"God made man to go by motives, and he will not go without them, any more than a boat without steam or a balloon without gas."
Henry Ward Beecher

Week Eleven, Thursday

Laughter

"Our mouths were filled with laughter, our tongues with songs of joy. Then it was said among the nations, 'The Lord has done great things for them.' The Lord has done great things for us, and we are filled with joy."
Psalm 126:1-3

We need to take laughter seriously. Really, we don't laugh enough. Everyone needs to laugh every day. Not only is it contagious but most certainly healthy. Laughing allows you to release tension, let your guard down, and elevates your psyche. Humor releases negative thoughts and patterns and replaces them with positive, elevated ones. Laughter breaks down walls. In Psalms we are assured that laughter can force the wicked, and thus Satan, far away.

It's true: he who laughs, lasts. The mind-body relationship of laughter and healing has been supported by medical research, signifying that laughter boosts the immune system. In 1964 Norman Cousins was diagnosed with ankylosing spondylitis, a degenerative disease of the connective tissue, and given only a few months to live. Cousins formulated that negative thoughts and attitudes can result in illness, and reasoned that positive thoughts and attitudes may have the opposite effect. So he left the hospital and checked into a hotel, took mega doses of vitamin C, and watched humorous movies and shows. Cousins discovered that ten minutes of boisterous laughter resulted in pain-free sleep for a minimum of two hours. He kept his routine until he fully recovered, proving that laughter is the best medicine.

We are reminded, however, that even in laughter the heart may ache, and joy may end in grief (Proverbs 14:13) and that sorrow is better than laughter, because a sad face is good for the heart (Ecclesiastes 7:3.) In these states, God desires to keep us close and we can choose to do the same.

Do you utilize humor to offset the havoc experienced in life's rigor? Does laughter offer balance and dissipate tension, anger, exasperation, fear, stress and depression? Does laughter allow you to see how God has richly blessed you?

"Laughter is the closest distance between two people."
Victor Borge

Week Eleven, Friday

Journey

"But he said to them, 'Do not detain me, now that the Lord has granted success to my journey. Send me on my way so I may go to my master.'"
Genesis 24:56

Perhaps you have applied justifications like *after this large project is completed . . . once everyone is healthy . . . when the kids get older . . .* and countless other reasons why utilizing back burners remains more convenient at this time than placing anything on the front ones. So you contrive the same list the following week, or the subsequent month, perhaps even the next year, hoping that your schedule eases a bit.

It rarely does. Each moment in the present is valuable. And while it is far more beneficial to be grounded in the present day than to be concerned with the future, it is vital to view each event as if tomorrow may not occur. Stay in the present moment, as tomorrow has not yet arrived and yesterday has already transpired. Presently enjoy the present. Recall the words of encouragement in Philippians 3:12-14, "Not that I have already obtained all this, or have already been made perfect, but I press on to take hold of that for which Christ Jesus took hold of me. I press on toward the goal to win the prize for which God has called me heavenward in Christ Jesus." Enjoy the untraveled earthly journey.

Could you accomplish your plan gradually, as you piecemeal the tasks? Is there room in your schedule to prepare for the event bit by bit, as a multitude of other incidents unfold in your life? Can you build upon your dream brick by brick, over time, starting today?

"There is meaning in every journey that is unknown to the traveler."
Dietrich Bonhoeffer

Week Eleven, Saturday

When the Sidewalk Ends

"He lifted me out of the slimy pit, out of the mud and mire; he set my feet on a rock and gave me a firm place to stand."
Psalm 40:21

Catherine's husband answered the call from her physician, sitting down as he listened intently. With fear taking over every fiber of her being, she solemnly looked at him, mouthing, *It's cancer, isn't it?*

She was thirty-seven when diagnosed with a fast-growing form of skin cancer. Despite the odds and the effects of surgery and chemotherapy, Catherine resolved to do all she could to keep her mind and spirit thriving and to achieve and maintain optimal physical health through diet and exercise.

Catherine focused on her plan daily as she exercised diligently, ate wisely, listened for God's voice, and loved her family and friends. Daily she set out on walks through the neighborhood, digital music player in position, setting goals with each step.

But one particular cold, icy day, Catherine couldn't find her portable media player. She set off without it, walking briskly and taking note of the sidewalk surfaces—some clear and some icy. On the icy patches, she slowed down. *Like unsteady episodes in life,* she thought, *when I am cautious,* and moved a bit more slowly through those spots. Other areas of the sidewalk had been shoveled, making faster walking safe and comfortable. *Like good times in life,* she thought, *when I am more carefree.*

As she walked, she also became aware of the dimensions of each square of sidewalk and the lines that separated them. *Like the steps in my life,* Catherine reflected. She had experienced so many new steps lately—surgeries, chemotherapy, hair loss, mood swings, despair. *But I am here today.*

Catherine continued walking until the sidewalk met the curb at an intersection. Panic set in. *What happens when the sidewalk ends?*

As she crossed the street, she was weeping. *Eventually I will have to cross over,* she realized. Catherine didn't realize it, but God was breaking through here.

Her mind raced with this reality until she entered the front door again, spotting the portable media player in clear view on the kitchen counter. *God must have wanted me to tune in to him today instead of the radio,* she thought.

Catherine's spirituality emerged more strongly with the advent of the cancer. She felt that she had a broken relationship with Christ. Was it fit for mending? Before her children were born, she had asked questions of her faith.

Now, in light of the circumstances, these questions had gained depth. What did she believe and stand for? Was it too late to put herself in line with God?

Few people go untouched by cancer. Perhaps you yourself have faced cancer, chances are, or know someone who is struggling with diagnosis and treatment. Possibly that person has already been taken by the disease. Yet cancer brought this woman to Christ. She found the hope she needed in her Savior to face the severe trial that had come her way. She found freedom even amid fear. She found that she could face each day, and each step of her daily walk, when she knew Jesus was walking with her. Christ is present for every trial—whether physical, financial, relational—or any number of other difficulties that come along in this broken world. In spite of difficult seasons, Christ has everything under control.

What trial do you currently face? What uncertainty weighs on your shoulders? Ask Christ Jesus to lift you from the pit of despair and to steady you as you walk along—today and every day—on a sidewalk that will not end.

> "Adversity has the effect of eliciting talents which, in prosperous circumstances, would have lain dormant."
> Horace

Week Eleven, Sunday

You Treasure, You

"For you are a people holy to the Lord your God. The Lord your God has chosen
you out of all the peoples on the face of the earth to be his people,
his treasured possession."
Deuteronomy 7:6

You are a treasure; a valuable fortune of the most high God. Launch this thinking in yourself daily as you live and believe it. First, accept who you are, flaws amid strengths, so that you can unreservedly accept others with genuineness and move into personal wholeness.

Once you reverentially accept yourself you can readily see areas in your life where you desire change. In order for change to be lasting, it needs to occur from within. Grow resiliently into completeness and your innate purpose, for to *not* follow your calling is literally, to weaken.

Are you an approval seeker? Examine your inhibitions, fears, and doubts. While we all desire to be loved and accepted by others at some level, suitable love and respect for ourselves equips us to pass it on. This is not composed of self serving, selfish, or self centered characteristics; rather it embodies healthy identity rooted in our Father's love for us. Our Creator fashioned us in His image. We can then alter our thinking to ask instead for His approval. Let us follow the narrow path He has set before us so that we may grow more Christ-like—the true fortune for the believer.

"Our deepest fear is not that we are inadequate. Our deepest fear is that we are
powerful beyond measure. It is our light, not our darkness that frightens us most
. . . You are a child of God. Your playing small does not serve the world . . . We
were born to make manifest the glory of God that is within us. It's not just in
some of us; it's in all of us. And when we let our own light shine, we
unconsciously give other people permission to do the same. As we are liberated
from our own fear, our presence automatically liberates others."
Return to Love by Marianne Williamson

Broken but Willing; Reduce and Grow

This Week

How God leads me . . .

_____
_____
_____
_____
_____
_____
_____

How I follow Jesus . . .

_____
_____
_____
_____
_____
_____
_____

How I hear the Holy Spirit . . .

_____
_____
_____
_____
_____
_____
_____

WEEK TWELVE

Aspire

to

Inspire

A time to be silent

and

A time to speak

Week Twelve, Monday

Move Like a Maverick

"Do not conform any longer to the pattern of this world, but be transformed by the renewing of your mind. Then you will be able to test and approve what God's will is—his good, pleasing, and perfect will."
Romans 12:2

    A maverick is a contrarian who travels opposite the trend. Mavericks can play by the rules and live with the norm until they realize that certain things have gone wrong. Without trying to be rebels for the sake of revolution, they see options. Altruistic mavericks realize that the change they seek will improve society. As a nonconformist who resists the norm, a maverick is a one of a kind thinker who steps forward with actions that create a stronger, better tomorrow—priceless when channeled in the right direction and for the greater good.
    When we reflect on personal growth and change ourselves prior to changing the world, we are better equipped to alter circumstances great or small. As soon as we wake each day, we have entered into change. Change is unavoidable. And our Heavenly Father is a God of change. Hence, He brought us the four seasons. He also brings us into and through circumstantial, chronological, and spiritual seasons.
    While adjustments are inescapable, growth is optional. We have choices greater than what to have for breakfast that place us at major crossroads for commitment. This cycle continues, no longer ordinary once we introduce transformation: aspirations, progression, and a future. Are you willfully moving in God's direction for you?

"Change is hard because people overestimate the value of what they have—and underestimate the value of what they may gain by giving that up."
James Belasco and Ralph Stayer from *Flight of the Buffalo*

Week Twelve, Tuesday

Believe with Certainty

"Jesus said, 'Don't be afraid, only believe.'"
Mark 5:36

My grandmother loved to bake. Each time I visited, it amazed me how she instinctually knew quantities and portion sizes from recipes etched into her memory. We kneaded and stretched dough, discussed life and faith. This drew me in—the comfort of baking and talking with someone who had experienced events I had not yet or perhaps wouldn't ever. Kind, loving, hard-working grandma endured hardships as a part of the overall plan—she had faith in a divine diagram that secured goodness, hope, and a future for all who had faith. In her words, *you have to have the faith.* What an inspiration.

Despite differing views and the imperfect world we live in daily, she chose a firm foundation: whole-hearted steady faith that God is alongside in all seasons. Just as grandmother knew with certainty the exact number of pinches and handfuls necessary for each recipe, she exemplified trust and a convicted life in what Christ-followers believe, even if not seen. Faith represents trust in the absence of fear. Believe that all things entail reverence and honor for each day that God made for you as you walk further along your faith journey daily.

How do you incorporate *don't be afraid, only believe* into your life? Do you allow doubt to creep into your thoughts? How can you avoid asking *what if* questions and escape the self-scare arena? Can you trust yourself and invite the Holy Spirit to control your life so that you can put fear aside, whole-heartedly working through those roadblocks that create fear?

"Fear imprisons, faith liberates; fear paralyzes, faith empowers; fear disheartens, faith encourages; fear sickens, faith heals; fear makes useless, faith makes serviceable."
Harry Emerson Fosdick

Week Twelve, Wednesday

Relinquish Your Burdens to God, the Beginning

"Come to me, all you who are weary and burdened, and I will give you rest.
Take my yoke upon you and learn from me, for I am gentle and humble in heart,
and you will find rest for your souls.
For my yoke is easy and my burden is light."
Matthew 11:28-30:33

I have lived through job loss and reduced business several times in my lifetime. In those seasons, God revealed to me that I needed to humble myself, trust Him, and not get ahead of the provisional and sequential seasons He had planned for me. During those times I found the following exercises helpful to relinquish my burdens to God.

Recognize self-defeating talk. Boost your self-confidence and self-esteem with positive messages. Realize that each and every glass is half-full, not half-empty. It's all good. Your attitude will rapidly match this uplifted talk.

Feel good about yourself. Don't take it personal, unless of course, you know you're responsible. Disappointments are a part of life. Learn to get up quickly after you fall. Everyone has some down days from time to time when they encounter obstacles. Channel these into opportunities. Feel valued—you are.

Lessen your load. Prioritize items requiring your immediate attention and ones that can wait. Delegate where possible. Learn to say "no" to events. Decelerate and truly enjoy the tasks at hand.

Overwhelming afflictions may seem disastrous to us, but to our Faithful Father they appear as minor details. Can you hand over just one burden to God today? Can you trust that He has the particulars covered? Are you visualizing more glasses as half-full?

"When you are down to nothing, God is up to something."
F.A.I.T.H.: Favorite American Inspirational That Helps

Week Twelve, Thursday

Relinquish Your Burdens to God, the Continuum

"Assemble the people—men, women and children, and the aliens living in your towns—so they can listen and learn to fear the Lord your God and follow carefully all the words of this law."
Deuteronomy 31:12

Script, sit, speak, or socialize—which one is appropriate for the troubled season you are in? Each situation is unique and warrants its own response. For instance, written and spoken words can be as powerful as reading someone's silence or sitting in silence. Find balance for well-being by practicing mastery over emotional reactivity, which will produce positive sentiment and sound health. The Holy Spirit has an opportunity to do work in your life when your approach is thoughtful.

Journal. Write it down. Place your thoughts, emotions, and feelings on paper. Journaling directs your inner energy appropriately. Reread your writing later, when you are in a fresh frame of mind. Re-write to train positive thinking.

Listen; then communicate. Voicemail, email, and text messaging complicate the communication theory. Ideally, listening intently while in the presence of another lessens the chances of missing important details and enhances our ability to see the other person's viewpoint. Effective communication and follow up decreases chances for misunderstandings, frustration, and avoidable stress.

Be assertive. Let your *yes* mean *yes* and your *no* mean *no* every day. Be proactive. Learn to ask for what you need. Take initiative. Be accountable. Socialize. While there is a place for solitude, regular connections are healthy. Socializing equates with a greatly fulfilled life and even a longer life. Social settings can consist of just you and a friend, or a grand party. Sharing events with others defrays stress and places life in perspective.

Can you carve out quiet time daily to journal and listen to our Mighty God's voice? Do you let your *yes* and *no* responses consistently equate to their actual implication?

"Don't speak unless you can improve on the silence."
Spanish Proverb

Week Twelve, Friday

Relinquish Your Burdens to God, the Finale

"Consider it pure joy, my brothers, whenever you face trials of many kinds, because you know that the testing of your faith develops perseverance."
James 1:2-3

These final points related to releasing your burdens to God also encourage you to indulge in blessings He has for you on earth. Prayer is forever at our core. Beginning and ending the day in prayer, and revering Christ prior to any thought or activity will change your latitude. Incorporate healthy lifestyle activities into your daily regimen such as:

Exercise. Whether you enroll in a yoga class, go for a walk during your lunch hour, or strength train with a friend, exercise decreases anxiety, increases muscular relaxation, and assists with a healthy balance. The natural endorphin release during exercise triggers our psyches into a "feel good" state.

Meditate. Be in the moment, and turn inward at least 15-20 minutes daily. Peace and solitude allow us to slow down and regain an optimistic outlook.

Breathe. Recognize that you are stressed when breathing is short and shallow. Slow down and lengthen your breath, taking eight counts to inhale and eight to exhale.

Pray. God meets you where you are. He also has a plan for how He would like you to grow—in His timing, not yours. It may seem that tackling milestones to arrive at the other side of the hill occurs frequently. Hill climbing tests our patience. We easily get frustrated, stressed, angered, and build up emotional resistance. Difficulties try our conviction. Prayer intervenes as trials test our faith, obstructing temptations. As a friend of mine says, ask Jesus to answer when Satan knocks at your door.

Which burdens have you relinquished to God this week?

"When we are sure that we are on the right road there is no need to plan our journey too far ahead. No need to burden ourselves with doubts and fears as to the obstacles that may bar our progress.
We cannot take more than one step at a time."
Orison Swett Marden

Week Twelve, Saturday

I Miss You

"I thank God, whom I serve, as my forefathers did, with a clear conscience, as night and day I constantly remember you in my prayers. Recalling your tears, I long to see you, so that I may be filled with joy."
2 Timothy 1:3-4

I miss you most when I've accomplished something that I didn't think I could do, and I long to tell you about it. You always made me feel special and confident. I miss you even more when thoughts plague me and concerns don't leave me, and I long to cry over it with you. You helped make sense of my disappointments and dissipate my fears. I miss you terribly when I want to hold your hand just one more time and it's not there. One thing I have learned very well: life is short.

With your words you closed up any disparity, assured me that differences in this world were intentional, and good. With your actions you showed me how to enjoy service to mankind and in the process exude peace, trust, and love. With your smile and that sparkle in your eyes, you told me *I love you* without uttering a word. Did I reciprocate for you? Was I there for you as you were each time to revived me?

I know that each encounter has been a part of me, impressed upon and shaped me. Show me, Lord, how to fill in earthly relational gaps, making them as close to whole as I can, like you always do with me. Teach me to recognize past shortcomings as future aspirations. Allow me to comprehend more each day, Lord God, that the relationship with you is supreme and that I long to see you once all my seasons have passed.

"Absence makes the heart grow fonder."
American Proverb

Week Twelve, Sunday

Seek Inspiration

"We continually remember before our God and Father your work produced by faith, your labor prompted by love, and your endurance inspired by hope in our Lord Jesus Christ."
1 Thessalonians 1:3

Some days I sit at my computer staring at the screen, waiting for inspiration to drop from the ceiling onto the keyboard. I won't claim "writer's block" since there is no such thing. A television repairman doesn't arrive at my home declaring, "Gosh, you know, I really don't feel motivated to fix your TV today; maybe tomorrow." Certainly we realize that inspiration is the flicker that leads to flames.

Fires start within. If somehow you've lost that burn, throw on a few logs and start up the bonfire again! The gumption resides in you. You say you can't remember what inspired you or how to get motivated again? Surround yourself with resources: rousing literature, tools and materials needed to further pursue your passion, and most importantly, encouraging, sagacious individuals who champion your cause.

Change the scenery. Think outside the box. Ask yourself, if you had all necessary resources available to you, what would inspire you? Extend your scope. Seek empowerment from the Source of all power, our omnipotent God. Be encouraged and follow your heart. Throw on the logs, light the fire, roll up your sleeves, and go for it.

"We are what we repeatedly do. Excellence, then, is not an act, but a habit."
Aristotle

This Week

How God leads me . . .

_____
_____
_____
_____
_____
_____
_____

How I follow Jesus . . .

_____
_____
_____
_____
_____
_____
_____

How I hear the Holy Spirit . . .

_____
_____
_____
_____
_____
_____
_____

Autumn

Revelation, arise
A harmonious concert
Opens performance

The tango of leaves
Vibrant colors encase time
And all fall in love

© Gabriella D. Filippi

WEEK THIRTEEN

Love

and

Be Loved

A time to love

and

A time to hate

Week Thirteen, Monday

Die to Live ~ Die to Love

"Like water spilled on the ground, which cannot be recovered, so we must die.
But God does not take away life; instead, he devises ways so that
a banished person may not remain estranged from him."
2 Samuel 14:14

If repairs were needed in my home I wouldn't ignore them and say that I was letting the house age gracefully, or that those aged parts to this old house would pull through on their own. Rather than allow framing to detach from doors or drains to remain clogged, hopefully I would take time to restore or replace what was necessary to have a fully functioning home. And if I needed assistance along the way, I would call upon family, friends, or professionals who could lend a hand.

In the same spirit, renewal takes time and support. A new start is often sought following successive winter seasons or having been knocked flat one too many times. Recovery in these instances may take a while in order to get back on both feet, to reality, in the groove. During this season, love and support from those who can pour into them are immeasurably necessary to carry them forward just one more day. Perhaps that person is someone you know. Maybe that individual is you.

Can you release the old, undesirable patterns and incorporate new ones that you have longed for and now grow to love? Can you allow yourself to be transparent in order to arrive at the core of your being ~ to permit the old self to pass away so that the new self, freshly rooted in Christ, is the lasting self continually growing closer to Christ? Can you allow the old self to die so that you can fully live and completely love?

"Being vulnerable doesn't have to be threatening. Just have the courage to be
sincere, open and honest. This opens the door to deeper communication all
around. It creates self-empowerment and the kind of connections with others we
all want in life. Speaking from the heart frees us from the secrets that burden us.
These secrets are what make us sick or fearful. Speaking truth helps you get
clarity on your real heart directives."
Sara Paddison, from *The Hidden Power of the Heart*

Week Thirteen, Tuesday

Agape as Your Guide

"By this all men will know that you are my disciples, if you love one another."
John 13:35

Agape is the Greek word for *loving with an open heart*. Christ's powerful devotion to mankind demonstrated agape love. Of all the instructions and directives we fulfill in life, love is the most powerful and important. With love we not only survive but thrive.

The wide open love of agape embodies heart, will, and intellect. Agape love is free, unrestricted, without guilt or gossip, nondiscriminatory, and self-sacrificing. Open love requires attentiveness, too. Once we love with an open heart it becomes clear that love is the most powerful means for conquering everything. Try it.

Author and speaker Leo Buscaglia's description of how to love like a young child embodies agape love:

"A four-year-old boy saw his elderly neighbor who had recently lost his wife, crying. The boy went into the old gentleman's yard, climbed onto his lap and just sat there. When he returned home, his mother asked what he'd said to the neighbor. The little boy said, *nothing. I just helped him cry.*"

Listen, hold, love. Be there. Love openly from start to finish one day. Then again the next. What responses do you elicit in yourself and others? How does loving with an open heart feel? How can you allow agape love to guide your steps throughout the peaks and valleys of each season?

"Love conquers all."
Virgil

Week Thirteen, Wednesday

Love More Today Than You Loved Yesterday

"Love must be sincere. Hate what is evil; cling to what is good. Be devoted to one another in brotherly love. Honor one another above yourselves."
Romans 12:9-10

We cannot survive in the fullest sense without love. Imagine if you and everyone you encounter spread tender words and actions, and the cycle continued? We would live in a fearless, considerate world. Fortunately, love is contagious.

Watch a child love. A child's love lacks doubt. It is simple, honest, and pure. When did we unlearn how to love like a child?

Love greater, deeper, stronger, longer. Deep-seated love lives outside of self. Love more people. Love more of life. Love more innocently. Love others as your Creator loves you with a steadfast love. How do we accomplish this task? Lasting changes typically occur slowly over time—"baby steps"—so tread one delicate step per day and cover a bit more territory every season.

Be a better spouse, partner, or friend. Take in more play time with your children, regardless of their age. Rekindle favorite memories with your siblings. Visit your grandparents, parents, aunts, or uncles more often. Tell people in your circle how much you love them every day. Invite your neighbor for tea, a meal, or just conversation. Teach your dog to play Frisbee. Climb a tree. Take in the sunset with a friend. Bear hug a loved one. Squeeze a hand. Smile at everyone you meet. Encourage, exalt, and enjoy everyone. Love deeply and with greater magnitude today than yesterday. Do this all while you still have the chance. This is your life. No regrets, right?

"The way to love anything is to realize that it might be lost."
G. K. Chesterton

Week Thirteen, Thursday

Love at the Core

"Love is patient, love is kind. It does not envy, it does not boast, it is not proud. It is not rude, it is not self-seeking, it is not easily angered, it keeps no record of wrongs. Love does not delight in evil but rejoices with the truth. It always protects, always trusts, always hopes, always perseveres. Love never fails."
1 Corinthians 13:4-8

Dr. Gary Chapman teaches us that there are five love languages which express our love and have us feeling sincerely loved in return: words of affirmation, quality time, gifts, acts of service, and physical touch. These verbal and non-verbal expressions maintain loving relations. Love is a choice and love makes the difference.

The ability to love, Dr. Chapman states, especially when you are not loved in return, can offer an incredible challenge. Christ's birth, life, death, and resurrection model this profoundly, and exhibit love to the core.

Love situated at our core can be our highest goal. As a brief exercise, place your name in each spot where "love" appeared in the 1 Corinthians verse above. Are you, or can you be, patient, kind, not self-seeking? Can you always protect, trust, hope, and persevere? Our Sovereign, Omnipotent, Prince of Peace does.

Knowing God then, we know love. To place love at the core of your existence requires an untiring commitment to the Giver of Life, with the belief that that through all seasonal situations love can triumph. This means that despite demands and accusations, complaints and battles, frustrations and disappointments, and all exhausted possibilities, love wins out. Have you tried placing love at the care for one? What does your day look like when you choose not to keep score?

"I have found the paradox, that if you love until it hurts, there can be no more hurt, only more love."
Mother Teresa

Week Thirteen, Friday

God's Amazing Love

"The Lord is my shepherd, I shall not be in want. He makes me lie down in green pastures, he leads me beside quiet waters, he restores my soul. He guides me in paths of righteousness for his name's sake. Even though I walk through the valley of the shadow of death, I will fear no evil, for you are with me; your rod and your staff, they comfort me. You prepare a table before me in the presence of my enemies. You anoint my head with oil; my cup overflows. Surely goodness and love will follow me all the days of my life, and I will dwell in the house of the Lord forever."
Psalms 23: 1-6

With certainty we know that each winter, buds remain buried underground awaiting their entrance above soil in spring; that the sun will rise every morning and set each evening; that if we visit a valley we will surely find lush vegetation and abundant development, just as we would witness a lack of flourishing growth at the mountain top. We can also be assured that no matter how many reside on earth God knows each and every one of us uniquely. How absolutely comforting, as the Psalmist David recites in this meditation prayer.

Allow God to show you His amazing love. Our El-Shaddai, God Almighty, restores us when we've had enough. He beckons us to take a break when the going gets tough. His omnipotence speaks to us as we face giants in our world. When we ask, He gives us what is appropriate. God's goodness reveals to us that even in our darkest hour, He provides us with over and above what we ever imagined.

We are grateful that in God's almighty act of love, he sent His son Jesus Christ for us to receive His never ending grace and mercy. Does love take on a more powerful meaning when woven into your life as the foundation of your faith? Are you accepting grace through God's love and the love you consequently sow into each moment?

"For I am convinced that neither death nor life, neither angels nor demons, neither the present nor the future, nor any powers, neither height nor depth, nor anything else in all creation, will be able to separate us from the love of God that is in Christ Jesus our Lord."
Romans 8:38-39

Week Thirteen, Saturday

Love at the Top of Your Life List

"I pray that according to the wealth of his glory he may grant you to be strengthened with power through his Spirit in the inner person, that Christ may dwell in your hearts through faith, so that, because you have been rooted and grounded in love, you may be able to comprehend with all the saints what is the breadth and length and height and depth,
and thus to know the love of Christ that surpasses knowledge,
so that you may be filled up to all the fullness of God."
Ephesians 3:16-19

If we desire more love, we need to be the ones who love more to begin with. If we desire kindness, we must be the ones who see opportunities for compassion and reach out first. If we desire change, we need to be the ones to make the initial modification. All facets of character point back to an intensity of love in life. Love more and receive more love.

We can reaffirm that as we know God, so we truly know love. You belong to God as creatures to their Creator, as property to its owner, as a bride belongs to her husband (1 Corinthians 6:19-20; Ephesians 5:25.) Take a few moments to contemplate love as your highest goal, centered at the core and fervently at the top of life's list.

Are you growing devotion to the characteristics that move you into a growth phase as you discard those qualities that you dislike in yourself—traits that keep you stuck. Are you, or can you be, patient? And can you be kind each day? Can you avoid gossip? Can you love more today than you did yesterday? Are you able to grow greater love into your personality, relationships, and life situations, while discarding portions that you dislike?

"Love many things, for therein lies the true strength, and whosoever loves much
performs much, and can accomplish much,
and what is done in love is done well."
Vincent van Gogh

Week Thirteen, Sunday

Love Throughout the Seasons

"Yet he has not left himself without testimony: He has shown kindness by giving you rain from heaven and crops in their seasons; he provides you with plenty of food and fills your hearts with joy."
Acts 14:17

Through each season we weather diverse conditions that test our character and refine our essence. We strive daily to rid ourselves of impurities and gravitate instead in the direction of traits that make us better. Hence, through each season there exists a time to lose and a time to gain, a time to hate and a time to love, a time to weep and a time to laugh.

The seasons recur year after year. When each year ends, we know that a new one filled with different opportunities and challenges is about to begin. As each season flows into the next, so too do our lives pass through seasons. We are born with a newness mirroring spring. We pass away with somberness, like that of winter. Our summer and autumn are the epiphany and culmination of all our learning experiences, year after year. We experience seasons in our daily lives, too, through seasons of sorrow and joy, pain and pleasure. When we are open to growth, we become seasoned as the seasons progress.

Have you witnessed God's love throughout the seasons? How are you experiencing God's love in each of your chronological, circumstantial, and calendar seasons as you grow spiritually?

"Go—grow—journey intently through the seasons of your life.
Experience fully, live passionately."
Gabriella D. Filippi

This Week

How God leads me . . .

_____
_____
_____
_____
_____
_____
_____

How I follow Jesus . . .

_____
_____
_____
_____
_____
_____
_____

How I hear the Holy Spirit . . .

_____
_____
_____
_____
_____
_____
_____

CLOSING MOMENTS

Seasons

A time for war

and

A time for peace

> "Be still and know that I am God."
> Psalm 46:10

He is. And He always will be. For everything there is a season that the *I am* has created. For every loss there exists somewhere a gain. For each tear shed, laughter subsequently awaits. For every moment of grief, a time of joy. For periods of devastation, restoration.

Be ready. Inevitably, unexpected accounts in our lives, the tumultuous seasons, throw twists and turns into our path. The various seasons in our lives edify that times of trial reinforce our need and even our desire for preparation. Earthly life exists as a preparatory school for eternity. While material possessions are replaceable, people are not. Life here is indeed short.

Perhaps there have been times in your life when you believe you have set brokenness in motion or damaged something beyond repair. The good news is that storms subside. The cross reminds us that we can rejoice when storms erupt; since we understand that God has bigger and better in store once they quiet down. Seasons allow us to seek repentance then celebrate His love for us. We can finally understand after falling so many times that life is what God intended it to be for us, and that through a humble nature we can grow closer to the Lord through Jesus, our source of soul peace. We can lay our concerns at the foot of the cross, lift them up into God's care, and ask for a pardon.

We acknowledge that war exists in the outer world just as it takes place inside us. Inevitably, the enemy waits while God prevails, as unexpected accounts in our lives throw twists and turns into our path. Yet we seek balance throughout life, in order to live harmoniously. Therefore, before we wage the external wars, God desires for us to resolve the internal battles that exist inside each one of us.

Rely on a grounding faith, which will forever offer guidance though every chronological, circumstantial, and calendar season. Anticipate God's guidance then as you enter each new Spiritual season, full of possibilities and opportunities for growth—and the possibilities are endless. Noteworthy episodes in life produce sorrow, joy, pain, and pleasure, much like the seasons in the year, presenting disguised opportunities called challenges. If you are open to growth, you will mature as the stages progress, to fully appreciate the four seasons of tribulation, anticipation, exaltation, and revelation. Winter complexities, spring opportunities, summer excitement, and autumn epiphanies comprise more than the calendar year; they make up your daily life and ultimately move you towards completion. Rest in Him each season. You will discover that through the seasons, you are seasoned.

There is a time for everything . . . This is yours.

Deliverance

The Prayer

Why not have a conversation with God, your Father, today? Let Him know that you confess that you have sinned against Him. Ask forgiveness for your sins. Ask Him to take over your heart. You are invited to recite this prayer:

Father, I know that I have broken your laws and my sins have separated me from you. I am truly sorry, and now I want to turn away from my past sinful life toward you. Please forgive me. Send the Holy Spirit to guide me, protect me, and counsel me. Protect me from Satan and his evil forces. Help me grow in wisdom, knowledge, and love for You and Your ways. Give me the strength and courage to change my ways and oppose sin in the future.

Lord, right now I accept Your only Son Jesus as my Savior and as the Lord of my life. I believe that Jesus Christ died for my sins, was resurrected from the dead, is alive, and listens to my prayer. I invite Jesus to become the Lord of my life, to rule and reign in my heart from this day forward. Lord, thank You for sending Your Son to die so that I can live. In Jesus' name I pray, Amen.

The Prayer of Salvation has three main parts:

Faith in God (Hebrews 11:6)
Confessing Our Sins (Romans 3:23; 2 Corinthians 4:6)
Professing Faith in Christ as Savior and Lord (John 1:1-3; John 3:16)

Allow Jesus to reign in your life from this day forward. Seek baptism as a seal of your new relationship with Christ. Spend time with God each day in prayer. Invite others to share your faith with you. Relationships add depth to life each season. Start with the most important relationship today: Christ the Savior.

> *Purposeful Relations and Experiences Add Depth To Life Each Season*

Soli

Deo

Gloria

Notes

Scripture quotations in this publication are taken from *the Holy Bible, Today's New International Version*^{TM} *TNIV* ®. Copyright © 2001, 2005 by International Bible Society. Used by permission—all rights reserved.

1. *Apache Seasons* used by permission from Manataka American Indian Council, Arizona, USA.

2. Lynne Giles and Gary Glonek, "Effect of social networks on 10 year survival in very old Australians: the Australian longitudinal study of aging," *Journal of Epidemiology and Community Health*, 2005; 59:574-579.

3. C. S. Lewis, *The Four Loves;* Orlando: Harcourt, 1991.

4. Richard Langworth (editor,) *Churchill by Himself: The Definitive Collection of Quotations;* Jackson: Public Affairs, 2008.

5. Ihaleakalá Hew Len, Ph.D., *Zero Limits: The Secret Hawaiian System for Wealth, Health, Peace, and More;* Hoboken: Wiley, 2008.

6. Martin Luther King, *Letter from Birmingham Jail.* Birmingham: Martin Luther King, Jr., April 16, 1963.

7. William A. Redding, *The Millennial Kingdom: A Book of Surprises Containing Unusual Statements Supported by Positive Testimony*; Kansas City: Hudson-Kimberly Publishing Company, 1894.

8. Norman Cousins, "Anatomy of an illness (as perceived by the patient)," *New England Journal of Medicine* 1976; 295:1458-63; "The Anatomy of Norman Cousins' Illness" (Kahn) *The Mount Sinai Journal of Medicine*, 1981; 48:305-314.

9. Williamson, Marianne, *A Return to Love: Reflections on the Principles of "A Course in Miracles;"* New York: Harper, 1996.

10. Henry Cloud, Ph.D. and Steve Townsend, Ph.D., *Boundaries: When to Say Yes, When to Say No, To Take Control of Your Life;* Grand Rapids: Zondervan, 2001.

11. Leo Buscaglia, Ph.D., *A Memory for Tino;* Thorofare: Slack, Incorporated, 1988.

12. Gary Chapman, Ph.D., *The Five Love Languages*; Chicago: Northfield Publishing, 2004.

Appendix
My Moments of Progression and Growth

A Time to be Born; a Time to Die

_____
_____
_____
_____
_____
_____
_____

A Time to Plant; a Time to Uproot

_____
_____
_____
_____
_____
_____
_____

A Time to Kill (do away with); a Time to Heal

_____
_____
_____
_____
_____
_____
_____

A Time to Tear Down; a Time to Build

_____
_____
_____

A Time to Weep; a Time to Laugh

A Time to Mourn; a Time to Dance

A Time to Scatter Stones; a Time to Gather Them

A Time to Embrace; a Time to Refrain

A Time to Search; a Time to Give Up

A Time to Keep; a Time to Throw Away

A Time to Tear; a Time to Mend

A Time to be Silent; a Time to Speak

A Time to Love; a Time to Hate

A Time for War; a Time for Peace

My purpose related to God's plan

My gratitude list

Author will donate a portion of all book sale proceeds to benefit Feed My Starving Children
www.fmsc.org

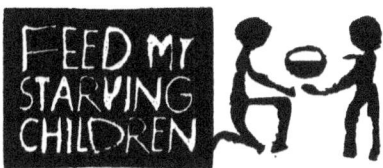

Little children let us love, not in word or speech, but in truth and action.
I John 3:18

Our Mission
Feeding God's Starving Children Hungry in Body and Spirit
Our Vision
With God's help Feed My Starving Children (FMSC) will strive to eliminate starvation in children throughout the world by helping to instill compassion in people to hear and respond to the cries of those in need.

From its beginnings, Feed My Starving Children (FMSC) has worked to develop a food mixture that would be easy and safe to transport, simple to make with only boiling water, and culturally acceptable worldwide.

With the input of scientists from major food companies, FMSC developed a formula packaged in small pouches—each of which provides six highly nutritious meals. This easy-to-prepare food blend has won rave reviews all over the world. While the formula was designed to save the lives of severely malnourished and starving children, the ingredients also improve the health, growth and physical well-being of children who are no longer in immediate danger of starvation. A team of food scientists continues to monitor the FMSC formula to ensure that it meets nutritional needs for the world's hungry children.

A single bag of food—which provides meals for six children—costs around $1 to produce, and 94 percent of all donations to FMSC goes directly toward the food program.

Blessed are those who are generous, because they feed the poor.
- Proverbs 22:9

Feed My Starving Children Headquarters
401 93rd Avenue NW
Coon Rapids, MN 55433
763.504.2919

Inspire me!

To obtain additional copies of

Celebrate Your Seasons

and to
Register for the newsletter visit

www.gabriellafilippi.com.

Receive motivation, encouragement, and news of upcoming events & appearances

**In search of more
Inspiration?**

Look for these
Upcoming releases:

Seasons
Sequel

and

Seasons
Inspirational Promise Box

www.ingramcontent.com/pod-product-compliance
Lightning Source LLC
Chambersburg PA
CBHW020746230426
43665CB00009B/527